Life after the Phone Rang . . .

Black & White Version

The step-by-step experience of

HER2-positive

hormone negative

Boob Cancer

Kaye Thomas

To my loving husband Jimmy.
Thank you for all your love, caring
and support through
this Speed Bump in life.
You are my rock and one
heck of a caregiver!

Thank you to my sister Lynne and
my granddaughter Aubrey
for proofing and pointing
out the errors!

To all my family and friends.
Thank you for your concern, prayers
and cheer.

The encouragement from everyone is part of the
reason I felt inspired to write this book.
Thank you,
Kaye

Dear Reader,

You may have just found out you have HER2-positive breast cancer and are feeling scared, worried or shocked. I can sympathize with every feeling you are having. Take a deep breath. Enclosed is the information I would have loved to have gotten when I was diagnosed with HER2-positive breast cancer. Read it and learn that this cancer is something you can beat! I have written this book for you, to give you what you need to feel empowered with information to handle the treatments, confidence to know that each step is progress and assurance that you can conquer this cancer while having a positive attitude, determination and humor.

I have three things I wanted to make sure I said to you.

First, I have written this book to give real information about what was my experience as the patient. I do not bore you with medical babble, you will get enough of that from the medical professionals! I have included only definitions to help you understand the tests and terms you may hear. The timeline on the back of the book is a visual for you to see the type of scheduling that will be part of your fight with cancer. Holidays can sometimes work in those breaks as you will see while reading about my experience. It will also give you and your caregiver an idea of what to be expecting and how to help you stay on schedule.

Second, to let you know that the pictures in the book were not taken for a book. What you see is what you get! The pictures are the reality of every step. Jimmy took the pictures for me to see the

—

difference in my hair growth, show family and to use on social media. The best thing was to see myself. My advice would be to do the same. Take pictures to show family and friends that you are getting the job done of fighting cancer. Take the pictures for yourself so that you can see your progress. Take the pictures to look back on what you went through and be proud. I look back at the pictures now and am so proud of myself. Yes, they aren't flattering, but they are reality. Reality of conquering boob cancer.

Third, I want to ask you a favor. While reading this book imagine that a dear friend is talking to you. A friend who is trying to help you prepare, understand, handle and complete a hurdle that you are not familiar with. If you would do this for me I have accomplished the reason for writing this book.

Thank you,
Kaye

Table of contents

Life before the Phone Rang
Chapter 1

Women go for mammograms or do the self-check every day.
A Mammogram is an X-ray picture of the breast using film. Most
women do not think anything of it, just one of those things that isn't
fun but part of being a woman. Thank goodness women now know
to feel for a lump or bump! I would stress young women should take
this seriously as this Breast Cancer is one that young women get.
The mammogram or the boob smasher session as I call it, is a
necessary part of being a responsible woman. Not that I have always
been a responsible woman.

My husband Jimmy and I have always had a very busy and
active life. We are proud parents of four children: Autumn, Aaron,
Austin and Amy, oldest to youngest. Jimmy worked as a
geologist/geophysicist and I stayed home to care for the kids. As I
would say when they were growing up, "name a stage and I probably
have one going through it." Any time-off from work and school we
spent with family. Many, many weekends at the family ranch,
fishing in Galveston and Palacios, vacations to Big Bend, New
Orleans, Corpus Christi and New Mexico. Our children are now full
grown with children of their own. We have quite a few

grandchildren and even two great grandchildren. Do not assume we are sitting in rocking chairs! Our life has always been full of family, work and each other. Like everyone else raising children, working and trying to handle daily struggles can be very consuming. To say the least there have been times I postponed being a responsible woman from time to time. Typically, it would be two or three years between the annual pap and mammogram.

We lived in Houston, College Station and at the ranch in central Texas while raising our family. Both Jimmy and I are from oilfield families thus we understood the roller coaster ride of the industry! The ups and downs could be dizzying at times, but we would always work our way through it. Like everyone else, there are times when the budget needed to be tightened and the kids need to know there would be some changes. One time as I talked to the kids about it while they were sitting at the dinner table and explained that we had to tighten our belts this month. I had the bills in a stack on the table. I picked up the stack and tossed them up in the air while saying, "we will pay the ones face up." The reaction of a slow-motion time in life happened. One that I wish I had recorded. Their eyes opened wide, and their mouths dropped as the bills landed on the floor. Autumn being about thirteen, was just getting interested in her hair style. She stood up and asked, "Is the electric bill face up?" Her hairdryer was the focus of getting dressed every day. I wanted to giggle but, I knew that they understood the lesson. Most of the time Jimmy's professional career involved being independent of any company. Austin born with heart issues, which made medical

—

insurance a must of the monthly bills. Even times when we had insurance I used the "I don't have time, life is so busy" excuse. I know that budgets get tight but, don't take being a responsible woman out of the budget. During my experience you would not believe how everyone we met wanted to know how the lump was found. I cannot remember how many times I was asked that question. Then they were amazed it was by a mobile mammogram unit. Do the research, there are places that offer free or minimal cost for a pap and mammograms. If we don't take care of ourselves, we may not be around for the family.

As time went on we were blessed that we didn't have any major medical issues. I did have endometriosis at one point. My pregnancy with Amy alleviated the endometriosis. Thank goodness Austin had his one major heart surgery at five months old. They operated with a new procedure that ended up keeping him from having surgery every four years as he grew. That enormous difference we learned to appreciate more as he grew up. Of course, we had the typical stiches, colds, ear aches, broken arm and smashed fingers. I never appreciated how often doors close on fingers! Austin and I happened to be the ones that a car door closed on our own fingers! Amy caught a finger in a heavy front door on the way out to collect chicken eggs, she closed the door herself too! Now, I am the over cautious Gammaw about the kids getting fingers caught in doors!

Our first encounter with cancer was Jimmy's parents. They both got cancer at the same time. Dad had stomach cancer and Mom

3

had hormonal breast cancer in the late 1990's. We lived at the ranch just down the road from them, thank goodness. Jimmy and I don't remember any details, except the port Mom had. Unlike the ports used today, hers was exposed and difficult to keep clean and open. I talk more about ports later in the book. She did have a mastectomy and chemotherapy and has been cancer free for twenty years! Dad ended up having his stomach removed and another created out of his intestine. He passed away from heart issues years later. Back then people didn't talk about what they experienced going through cancer. Most of the time you may or may have not even known when someone had cancer. Even now with the many advances they have made with cancer many people don't generally talk about the process of fighting cancer and all that it involves. There have been many changes in the information available on cancer, chemotherapy and radiation. It is now a subject you can easily get information of on the internet, but the data is quickly outdated, and some is erroneous. Now there are people, like me who want to tell their story and pass on helpful information and encouragement on how to help with the process of fighting cancer. Talking about it in the open is one of the first and best steps!

As time went on and the kids grew into adults we had them leaving home for work or college. When our first, Autumn departed, I swore I was not going to cry. As she left the driveway to move to Colorado I burst into tears. Damn, it is hard being a Mom even when they are grown! Aaron got married and at the wedding I couldn't believe how I couldn't stop the tears again! Austin was his groomsman and had trouble not crying too. I kept looking at him and tried to be strong. So much for that! Austin got married, before the wedding I had convinced myself that I had done this and determined not to cry. Wrong! Here came the fountain of tears. Autumn got married, tears were abundant! Next Amy, our last to get married, Amy took a year to plan her wedding, so I felt empowered it was to be the exception! Wrong Again! Some things never change, like being a Mom.

We lived in Corpus Christi, Texas at the time and all the kids lived there too. Having the kids, grandchildren, my sister Lynne, nieces and nephews around to make many memories. When we moved to Corpus Christi I had decided to become a very responsible woman. I had a General Practitioner and a Gynecologist, went to regular checkups, annual pap and mammogram. In the beginning, I did very well for about five years. During that time, I had only had one mammogram that showed some tiny calcium deposits that looked like the Seven Sisters constellation in my left boob. Life got hectic and I fell into the old rut of too busy.

We woke up the morning after returning from a trip when my sister Lynne called. She said that she had been ill and needed help. Jimmy and I rushed over to her house to be shocked at how very ill she had become. Lynn said that she thought she had the flu. She had become so weak, and it hurt for us to touch her. Obviously, she needed to go to the emergency room. Just lifting her in the car, in the wheel chair and on the bed, she experienced excruciating pain. Within hours they moved her to a room, started blood tests and gave her saline as she was very dehydrated. We had just gotten her to a room when she told me "I can't breathe, I feel like I'm dying!" I ran out to the hall yelling "She can't breathe! Help! She can't breathe!" The staff came running to her room. One nurse asked me to wait in the hall while what must have been four nurses and two doctors helped her. They intubated Lynne and took her to the Intensive Care Unit. Lynne and I said in our younger years, "It's us against the world." Our father died when we were in our very early twenties and our mother diagnosed with Alzheimer's in our late twenties. Most of our adult life we have lived near each other.

They ran every test known to man. The doctors tried to keep her body balanced. Her little body reacted in so many ways. At one point the doctor told us that anyone that wanted to see her needed to come. I kept talking to her, telling her to fight, she had so much more living to do. At one point I told her she can't leave me, "I am the oldest, I am supposed to go first!" After thirteen days they had to remove the breathing tube or do a tracheotomy because extended time on a ventilator will cause permanent damage to the vocal cords or windpipe. Once they removed it, Lynne began breathing on her own and regained consciousness within hours. She awakened very confused as to what had happened. At that point her body decided to start cooperating and responding. Lynne is so funny, one time while sitting in ICU with her just chatting. Jimmy had left to give us some time together. Within minutes Lynne put out her hand like she wanted to hold my hand. When I took her hand, she said "Pull!" Lynn wanted me to take her out of there! The fighter in my sister was back! They never did figure out the cause, only that her body started fighting back. She had to go to rehabilitation to learn to walk again and build her muscles. To this day you would never guess what she went through. I think it is the fighter in her that had to wake up and take charge! I thought of Lynne's battle when I was diagnosed, that her spirit had to fight. I know that's true, I had seen it. This experience is one I learned from and used in my battle with breast cancer.

Once we knew Lynne had gotten back on her feet, then began the question of "is it time to retire?" We were not sure where we wanted to retire to. It is amazing how through the years while raising kids couples have conversations of what they will do when they retire. Interesting how those thoughts may not be what you want when you finally reach that point in decision making. Traveling is part of what we wanted to do, but where to have home base had be decided first. We had several possibilities in mind. Traveling after the kids were grown had been a blast. We had our favorites! After lots of research and trips to check out areas we had pretty much decided to be in the mountains. At the time we lived in Corpus Christi, Texas, a coastal city, so that meant a big move! This all sounds well and good. On the third try Jimmy was ready to retire. I thought my life had been busy raising four kids, starting retirement is like bungie jumping. You make a decision, then spring back to the logistics of what must be done. As you might guess, being a responsible woman got put on hold. I just kept putting it off, too much to do. Don't have time.

—

7

Years ago, we had purchased a house in Alpine, Texas, a family favorite of places to visit. We planned on selling it and buying our retirement home. After all the research and trips to look at other areas we realized Alpine had all we wanted and necessary to retire. In the end we realized that we could remodel the house to create Our Home. The beginning of the remodel started, and it became obvious we needed to be nearby, so we took our 5th wheel to Lajitas to stay in for what ended up being six months. Our daily schedule consisted of going to the house to answer questions about the remodel. Return in the evening to discuss changes or order specific materials. The crew working on it were fantastic. They became close friends of ours. We had our house in Corpus Christi on the market. Everything running smoothly to the parking point. This is when I thought that I should be responsible and get that mammogram done before we moved and changed doctors. I made the appointment, it had been five years! Time had flown by without my noticing!

The week before my mammogram appointment, our youngest son Austin died from a heart aneurysm. His death was unexpected, in fact Austin had an appointment with his cardiologist the next week. During that dreadful day Jimmy, Aaron and myself had tried to get ahold of Austin. We called the RV park he lived in to see if the office would walk over to his trailer to let him know we were trying to reach him. Austin worked as a landman in the Midland area. They said there had been no response to knocking, just heard the dogs bark. They would not force the door to get in, so

Aaron called a friend in the area. His friend went to the trailer and forced the door open to find Austin dead on the floor. The Sheriff called us and immediately asked if Austin had heart problems. As part of procedure when a young person dies at 29 in Texas there is an automatic autopsy. Evidently Austin had taken a hot shower and it had caused the aneurysm to burst. We left immediately to Big Springs where Austin lived. Jimmy is my rock. Jimmy made the necessary phone calls while I just sat in shock on the drive. When we got to the hotel I kept looking out the window wondering where they had taken Austin. The only feeling at that moment reminded me of getting to hold him like I did when at five months old and he had come out of heart surgery. The nurses instructed me to sit in a rocking chair and laid Austin in my arms with all the wires and IV's. At that moment I just wanted to hold my precious son. I felt like the world turned upside down and helpless.

Austin had a very warm-hearted soul. To this day I can hear him coming in the door saying, "Hi Momma!" arms open for the hug. From the day of his birth Austin did everything early, he started talking at nine months! He woke up every day as a child smiling and living each day like an adventure. The loss of a child is devastating. My head and heart mourned for close to three years before I could fathom getting back to doing the normal things.

This experience also helped to keep being told I had breast cancer in perspective. We all have these kinds of experiences, use them.

In the two and half years since Austin's death we had sold

—

our house, moved into our home to retire in, settled in and were beginning to try to live again. That also included being a responsible woman. I found a new doctor, made the appointment for a general checkup and set an appointment for a mammogram. We live in a small town so there is a mobile mammogram unit that comes around every six months. The unit had just been in town, so my boob smasher session would be five months away in January of 2017.

When I got the mammogram done it had been eight years from my last one. After the boob smasher session, I went home for my relaxing afternoon cup of coffee, when the phone rang.

Stop the Head Spinning!
Chapter 2

The doctor wanted me to go back and have more pictures taken at the mobile mammogram unit. I have implants and had those few small calcium deposits before, so I thought nothing of it. That is the Pollyanna Positive in me as my family likes to call it. When I got the second call from my doctor, they needed to schedule a diagnostic digital mammogram and ultra sound in El Paso. A Digital Mammogram is when X-rays are used to produce detailed images of the breast using a digital receptor and computer. An Ultrasound (also called Sonography) is the use of sound waves to record the echoes as the waves bounce back to determine the size, shape and consistency of soft tissues and organs. They told me the nurse would make all the arrangements. First question, who would take my insurance, who my insurance would accept? Then they had to have the records from Corpus Christi before they would make an appointment. By May, four months had passed and still no appointment. I don't know if that four months made a difference, it did not help to think about that. The point I would press is if there is anything showing up on a mammogram, move on it, make it happen. If you are lucky enough to catch the tumor early, it could be non-invasive or in situ carcinoma. (*in situ is when the cancer is in its original place, not spread*) It means it is encapsulated and has not invaded the normal tissue. You can stop the cancer before it is a strong threat to your body and the treatment is simpler and less aggressive. In situ is very important, stop it before it escapes!

Then a few days later we made an appointment with my doctor to get the ball rolling. Within days we traveled to El Paso to get the next pictures of my right boob. The next phone call came with the report, a 1.9-centimeter mass that was consistent of invasive ductal carcinoma, which meant that the cancer has spread to the surrounding breast tissue. We made an appointment to have an ultrasound-guided biopsy. It is very simple and quick. During the procedure and while doing the biopsy they placed a titanium clip, which as the protocol at the time. During my treatment, a new pin became approved to be put in during biopsy that would have saved having the placement before surgery. We were told the results would be available in four to five working days. After that we referred to it as a Lump.

Our nerves did get twitchy for Jimmy and I waiting for the results of the biopsy over a three-day holiday weekend. Pollyanna Positive kept saying "I am sure it is nothing." During the waiting time we celebrated our 36th anniversery. As hard as that might be able to do, we decided that we would not talk about probable breast cancer that day. We had a wonderful day and a romantic dinner with my favorites, steak and asparagus! Days later we called to see if the results had come in, the doctor said the lump in my right breast was malignant. He wanted us to come in that afternoon to explain the results and help get us started on our journey.

Let the Head Spinning Begin!

We were at the beginning of June. I know now that I heard everything the doctor said about the results. The only problem is it went in one ear and right out the other. If I have learned anything, get a paper copy so you can read it later and take someone with you for a second pair of ears. I have always thought any time you go to the doctor, take someone to listen as the patient does not always hear what the doctor says or hears only what they want to hear. It is also good to have someone ask questions that the patient does not realize needs to be asked. My results came back as Invasive HER2-positive, Stage 3, hormone negative carcinoma. What we later learned was the cancer had left the tumor into the surrounding tissue. The English language used for medical information was still medical babble to us as we had no experience or knowledge of the types of breast cancer. Jimmy and I have always been healthy, nothing very serious. We had his parents that had cancer, but did not really know much about it. As I have said it is a subject people with cancer do not talk about it enough for others to understand.

We went back home both speechless. Your head starts spinning because of your imagination and ignorance creating a kaleidoscope of emotions. It is hard to stop, but you must take control of your emotions to begin gathering information. Do not panic!

The results from the biopsy was the information my oncologist needed to get the ball rolling in order to put together the team and protocol needed to tackle the cancer. There are three receptor indicators; estrogen, progesterone and a protein called human epidermal growth factor receptor 2 (HER2). If you really think about it breast cancer is a group of cancers. The results from my biopsy were negative on estrogen and progesterone, positive for HER2. HER2 is the protein that causes breast cancer cells to grow and can cause aggressive breast cancer. HER2-positive is said to be a more aggressive cancer compared with hormone positive cancers and triple negative cancers. The word "aggressive" did not even register to me. Pollyanna Positive kept saying "This cancer is not more aggressive than me!" There are many types of breast cancer, all have different protocols. HER2-positive is not like the other breast cancers. In the past it has been one of the most difficult cancers to help women survive. With the medical discoveries it is now one that can be cured. I will be telling the story of my journey with HER2-positive. I could not help but think about the name as Her Too! It is like being picked for a team in a game that I had not planned on playing.

There is no time for Lollygagging! Getting information on your insurance is first and foremost to make the decision of where to go for treatment. If you don't have insurance, there are many organizations that can help with information and funding to help with the cost. One example in Texas is the Susan G. Komen® organization. We started calling around before checking insurance, that is a waste of time. The insurance coverage had several options for me as we live far away from a large city in Texas. So much has changed in the cancer treatment world. When we lived in Houston it had become well-known for being the place to go for cancer. There are treatment centers everywhere compared to long ago when Houston was the only option in Texas. My doctor referred us to doctors in Austin with the Austin Cancer Center. The doctors and staff are the most attentive, caring and personal people I have ever met in the medical field. Even in the cardiology field with Austin as a baby, it lacked the genuine sensitivity. Our relationship with them has been a big part of feeling positive.

Next is the beginning of the Information Folder. Jimmy took charge of the paperwork. I strongly suggest starting a folder to put everything in. Jimmy is a wonderful caregiver, he kept on top of all the paperwork, billing, insurance, appointments and all that entails. We are retired so a work schedule did not need to be considered. In fact, we felt blessed that this happened at a time we could take a year to handle it to the best of our abilities. If you work, I have heard that many employers will work with you during your treatment. After my experience I would assume you will need more flexibility with work towards the last half of chemotherapy. In our case we had to plan on staying near Austin. Our home being over 400 miles away from Austin did not work. In fact, my doctor did not feel comfortable with me being that far away. Thankfully we had the house at the ranch that we had lived in while raising the kids to park while in treatment which is one of the reasons for choosing Austin. It was only 80 miles to see the doctor, hospital and less for some of the testing and radiation.

At the middle of June, the meetings were set up with the different doctors. We set out to Austin to be there for the meetings without any idea of our schedule, how much to pack for how long and didn't prep our home for being gone long. Now began the reality of the cancer and the plan. The first appointment is with the surgeon. As she spoke I heard lumpectomy. It was exactly what Pollyanna Positive had told the kids! "No problem probably just be a lumpectomy."

Next appointment, my oncologist. As he spoke I heard chemotherapy and hair loss. Anything else he said went in and out of my head. He gave us so much more information that Jimmy heard for me. Thank goodness.

There went the Head Spinning with a touch of shock! The amazing part is the small size, I had looked on a ruler. How could something so small take so much to kill it? The time of an entire year too! I felt emotionally dizzy. We got to the car and I broke out in an unusual outcry of curse words. Damn it! Pollyanna Positive's prediction had been only partially correct! The lumpectomy would be AFTER chemotherapy. I am not known for emotional outburst, but, it ended up being one of the healthiest things I did that day. To get the emotions of being frustrated, angry, pissed and disappointed that this was not going to be a quick and easy fix. Not just an operation or a pill to make this go away. Now is not the time for Whining, just action!

Jimmy had been terrified it would kill me, but after all this additional information and explanation sunk in we both realized that in this fight Boob Cancer had the odds stacked against it! It would not beat me. This is just another Speed Bump in our life. The doctors said that the timing of getting HER2-positive had really become a good breast cancer, if there is such a thing. The new specific medicine worked very well at attacking it. Up to recently HER2-positive had been known to be a more serious breast cancer. The new medication is trastuzumab (Herceptin®), has increased survival rates for women with stage 1 to 3 HER2-positive breast cancer by more than 30%. The technical diagnosis on my record of HER2-positive stage 3 became more understood for us.

Stage 0: Carcinoma in situ (not spread) – Early form

Stage 1: Localized

Stage 2: Early Locally Advanced

Stage 3: Late Locally Advanced

Stage 4: Metastasized

Thank goodness it waited to pop its ugly head up now. The acronym is HER2, I couldn't help but to keep writing Her Too! It is aggressive and had already left the tumor. There was no way to know if it had made it to the lymph nodes.

It is not hereditary! That was a relief for my girls!

I felt sad about the hair loss. My long beautiful hair that went down to the small of my back. The hair that Jimmy loved, that I loved. This immediate reaction is shared by almost every woman I have talked to who had breast cancer. I kept saying "Oh my, I am going to miss my hair."

Then the realization of no hair verses life, no question, hair will come back. New hair might be very interesting! Jimmy explained how he thought I should cut it in stages to get accustomed to it and make it less traumatic. His idea helped in so many ways! My caregiver had suggested what would be best for me already! I shared my missing hair adventure with family and friends on Facebook.

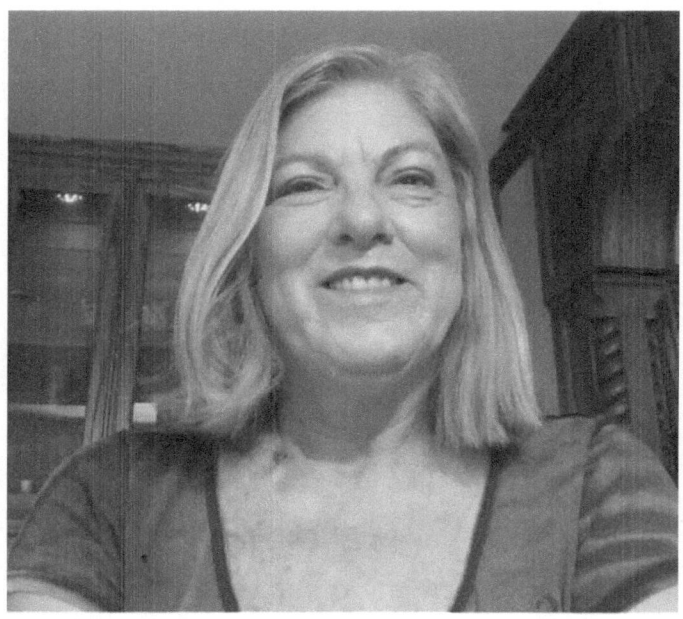

I cut off 12 inches to my shoulders and got use to brushing less hair. I even got to liking it and playing with it. This length I knew would be in my future so why not experiment now!

Preparing for the next step we picked out a cute pixie cut for after I had my first chemotherapy infusion. Jimmy bought me a cap with a wig attached for when my hair ran away. We did buy a couple of wigs and a partial wig but, the cap with the hair ended being my favorite. I kept using it constantly, partially because of the ease to grab and put on. I did try wearing funny and cute hats given or lent to me from family but that did not work for me like I thought it would.

The next step involved meeting with my radiation oncologist. He explained that I would receive the radiation after chemotherapy and surgery. He would have the before and after images that would be used to decide my radiation treatment. The radiation oncologist said that by the time I would be getting my treatments there would be a new machine and new treatment that I might qualify for. Another improvement during my protocol. After meeting with all the doctors in one week we immediately began scheduling all the testing needed before the chemotherapy began. A few days later for what seemed like a long week, we were going to get an MRI, EKG and PET Scan. These tests are not done at the cancer center. We used our GPS as we ended up going all over Austin! What an immense help. There is also a nurse coordinator that helped with trying to work with us several times in the beginning. If you need information or have a question the nurse coordinator can be very helpful. She helped us coordinate getting these tests done.

First the MRI it is Magnetic Resonance Imaging in which scanners use magnetic fields, electric field gradients and radio waves. EKG or ECG is the recording of the electrical activity of the heart over a period using electrodes on the skin. PET Scan is

Positron-Emission Tomography where a small amount of radioactive tracer is given through a vein inside the elbow to look for disease in the body. There is a one-hour wait in a cold room before they can do the scan. You wait in the cold room, I mean Cold room! I would recommend taking a jacket and they will offer blankets while you wait too.

All the technicians and nurses were very helpful and great at explaining every step. The tests are not scary, and they do not hurt, just tiring running around Austin and keeping the schedule. The insurance rejected some of the tests. Advice about insurance denying services: Don't freak out! Many of these denials are handled by the doctor by a peer-to-peer review. Let the doctors and center handle it. Insurance is so much faster and up-to-date with everything being done electronically now.

Next to have the port surgery. The Port is a small medical appliance installed with surgery beneath the skin. A catheter connects the port to a vein. They gave me a rubber bracelet to wear to alert medical staff that I had a Port. It is reassuring in case we had been involved in a car accident. Women who had ports used for chemotherapy years ago said the port had been a hassle, they were evidentially exposed, quite hard to maintain and subject to infection. The ports used now are wonderful. I would highly recommend one if your doctor suggests it. I do not know what the qualifications are for a port. My first impression is that some chemotherapy medications can only be given through a port, because they are too harsh or caustic to use an IV to the vein. One other possibility may be poor veins. The port is placed under the skin a couple of inches below your breast bone. It literally feels like a small rubber ball just under the skin that they insert the IV for infusion. The best part is that they can take blood and get the infusion with one needle prick. The port is a day surgery. I had no issues. They say you can start Chemotherapy even the day of the surgery. I had a week before infusion, extra time for the incisions to heal. Now I have the tools and tests done to start Chemotherapy!

The reason I call it "Boob Cancer" instead of "breast cancer," is it diminishes the disease. What a foolish disease that doesn't know it can't win against me! This is the point when I realized that I was not scared! Fear had not in any way entered my thoughts or heart. I knew that I had to convey this to Jimmy and the kids. They had to feel it too. Attitude is a huge part of defeating cancer and the phases of treatment. Attitude is key as most doctors will tell you! A positive, dedicated attitude will be your edge on cancer.

We had the appointment for the first infusion set. We had explained that we needed a week to go home to prep the house, get clothes and things needed for staying an extended period of time.

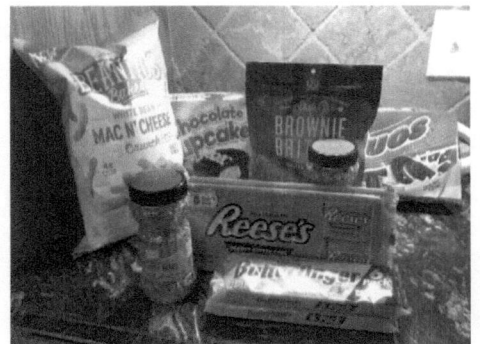

Autumn had flowers (pink roses) and treats for me in the house when we got in! I love her thoughtfulness!

While home we had planned that Autumn would be helping with the mail, etc. Aaron had mowed my precious back yard! Our friend Glen had weeded and trimmed everything in my back yard. It is not very big, but it is full of the plants, flowers and rocks under very tall trees. My little piece of heaven just outside my back door. The kids were worried, I hoped to ease their minds by coming in and showing them my determination and positive outlook! It would be good to let the kids see Momma in a "fighting hard" mode. They have seen me when I am determined to accomplish a task! With this visit home they knew we had prepared ourselves to rock this mission! "Imagination" and the "unknown" for family can create horrible images, paint a worse picture and wrong conclusions. Keeping family informed is much better than them guessing. It also gives you an opportunity to show them how to handle something in life that is not planned. Cancer treatment is now your Job!

We went back a couple of days before the scheduled infusion. Jimmy wanted to get back to clean the house before treatments started. He even detailed my Land Cruiser! It hadn't looked that clean in years! He shampooed the carpet! My SUV is my baby. It is my favorite vehicle ever and I plan on driving her till the wheels fall off and the engine falls out!

I felt for Jimmy, he is so wonderful, helpful and considerate! This would be hard on him and for an entire year. I couldn't help but hope and try to breeze through it. I could not imagine that going through this physically could be worse or as bad as losing Austin. I could not be weakened again emotionally like

---

that, hence the positive attitude and attitude of being tough physically! I also could not help but be glad that I had been the one that developed cancer. If this checks it off the list for us, I would much rather it be me and be Boob Cancer. I know that we will have other issues as we get down the road, but this Speed Bump has spikes if you back up! I also kept thinking it would be like Mononucleosis. I had Mononucleosis at about sixteen. I had it bad enough that the doctor put me in the hospital. My memory is mostly of not being able to even stand up long enough for a chest x-ray and them constantly feeding me steak and ice cream. Mono symptoms and lose my hair. I am good with that!

It had been so refreshing to be home and seeing the kids! I felt ready to get going with the chemotherapy but had enjoyed this bit of freedom before it started. Kept thinking if I could just stay long enough for July 4th Fireworks from my front porch, I know it sounds silly, but it is always so beautiful, it would be great if I could. Facts are we needed to get back and get rocking. After that trip home the kids felt confident that the outcome would be good, and we felt recharged to begin.

Chemotherapy Preparedness
Chapter 3

Your treatment is guided by the protocol for your cancer type. Protocol is the agreed precedence for the treatment needed that has been set by the medical community from their research. Our Doctor told us that if I got all the treatments in the protocol that our chances of beating the cancer would be very good. The caregiver's job is to try to help the patient stay mentally and physically healthy so that all treatments could be done without interruptions. The protocol for HER2-positive is six chemotherapy treatments, surgery, radiation and only the Trastuzumab (Herceptin®) infusions in the final stretch. As I mentioned earlier, there are various kinds of breast cancers therefore there are different protocols for each breast cancer. Time between my chemotherapy treatments was 3 weeks. Part of the caregiver's job is to help keep the patient on track for the chemotherapy treatments. The caregiver helps with encouragement, food preparing and just being there.

Jimmy was anxious to see that there were no hitches while we were going through this. He changed the oil and put new brake pads on my Land Cruiser. It is like planning a wedding. Plan the best you can and look for the one thing that will happen and get past it! Pollyanna Positive kept saying "It won't be as bad as you can imagine." She is always there to help me keep the good attitude I need!

Jimmy prepped the house for chemotherapy. He cleaned it from top to bottom to start as germ, dust and dirt free as possible. I don't think the floors were ever that clean when we lived there! Jimmy changed out all the filters, dusted, washed sheets and bleached the bathroom. The house smelled clean as a hospital but better with scented disinfectant! A caregiver is a Powerful help, especially one like Jimmy! He created a "bubble" for me to help with my white count down the road. The ranch is in the middle of nowhere. It is very wooded, lots of wild life, including deer, bobcats, snakes (*I hate snakes*), armadillos, opossums, raccoons, foxes, skunks and many varieties of birds. The closest neighbor is miles away. At night it is the meaning of Dark! This was going to be a bubble that could not be popped!

It had just begun, and I felt touched by the work and thought that he did to get ready. We also strongly recommend a good GPS for your vehicle, especially if you are getting your treatments and testing in an unfamiliar city. During everything we experienced this was an essential element of dealing with driving all around Austin. We had two pets that came along with us. Our faithful Yorkie, Phoebe was familiar with the ranch. She worships the ground Jimmy walks on and will follow him anywhere. I am just a part of the herd and her car seat. The ranch is her favorite place, it has lots of stickers, scorpions and cows that she likes to chase. As long as she is with us she is happy. Our other pet is my sugar glider, Quigley.

25

Jimmy had purchased another cage for when we went to the ranch with him. Little did we know how much time he would be living in it! The efforts needed for me to stay clear of dirt and germs meant Jimmy had to be in full charge of the pets. Watching Jimmy develop his relationship with my sugar glider kept me giggling every day. His connection with Quigley created a new regularity of laughter at feeding time. Jimmy ended up giving him a nickname, Buzzard Billy. The nickname stuck!

In the mean time, I made sure I had comfortable clothes with open necklines for infusions and comfortable but not sloppy clothes for wearing around the house. I knew that I might not be feeling pretty but I sure as hell would not stop trying!

Everybody in your family and your friends need to know that you will not be able to be as involved or helpful during the coming year. There won't be any dropping by to visit, there may not be long phone calls or any ability to help as you might normally do. It is a time to minimize life lists to keep focused on the battle of cancer. This may sound cold, but, your energy needs to be used for getting through all the steps of your protocol to beat cancer. If you or your caregiver need help, ask for it. Let those who care know you will call if needed. Just assure them you are doing everything you need to do to be around for a long time.

The team of doctors will usually provide a booklet or binder with information on where to call after hours, what is suggested for certain side effects, nutrition and even recipes. Keep it handy! Next, we gathered supplies to help handle the side effects. The information on side effects is not something that is a focus of the medical team I think because they do not know your bodies reaction yet. Looking it up on the internet can be disastrously wrong. A possible dilemma is the beginning of a side effect that begins at midnight and you are not near a store or the stores are not open! One of the things that I hope by writing this book is to help with an idea of what might be needed for chemotherapy. This is a list compiled of the things I needed during my chemotherapy. Talking with the other patients on different protocols it would have helped them and often did help them too. As always check with your doctor before taking anything, even over the counter! They want to make sure it won't interfere or have a reaction to anything involved in your protocol. If you are the patient, caregiver or want to help someone starting chemotherapy just getting a container of the basics can be a huge convenience for them when a side effect starts without warning.

Chemo Care Basics Basket
Be prepared for the onset of a side effect anytime of the night or day!
(Generic is cheaper on all these items)

Lotion for your skin (light or no fragrance)

Anti-diarrhea (Imodium® - loperamide hydrochloride)

Vitamin A & D® Ointment (for rashes)

Mild Laxative

Gas Relief

Antacid (Pepto Bismol®)

Lip Balm

Antacid chewable tablets (Tums®)

Salt (for salt water to rinse your mouth or brush your teeth)

Lemon Tea (for digestive irritation)

Hand Sanitizer (without fragrance)

Peppermints

Baby powder (for rashes)

Disposable gloves

Calamine lotion (for rashes or itching)

Chemo Care Big Basket
(get a bigger basket and add these items to the basics)

Pedialyte® (Electrolyte solution) and/or Sports drink

Bouillon

1 to 1 ½ Band-aids (for sores, boils, etc.)

Triple antibiotic ointment (for sores, boils, etc.)

Hydrocortisone cream (for sores, boils, etc.)

Hydrogen peroxide (for sores, boils, etc.)

Saline nasal spray (to moisten nasal passages)

When needed these items will be priceless! Adding a favorite food would always be appreciated. Jimmy always brought me "prizes" during chemotherapy, he out did himself. Remember during chemotherapy there will be cravings, only certain foods and flavors are appealing. When helping someone on chemotherapy ask if there is anything you can get for them that they are wanting, or just needing can be a wonderful treat or very helpful.

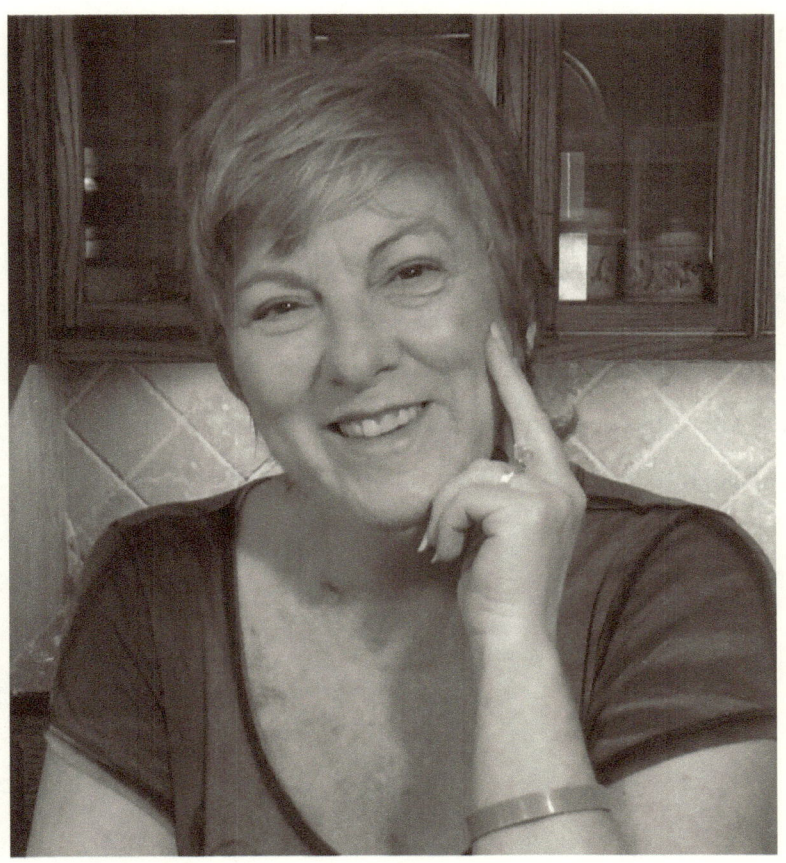

Just about ready to start, now for the next haircut into a pixie. My hairdresser did an excellent job and offered to shave my head when the time came. The shortness of my hair with the new haircut did feel like wearing a wig!

At this point I was not nervous about treatment. Ready! Curious how the effects will be. I could not imagine being extremely sick. I was concerned about how it would affect Jimmy. He was concerned, and I think nervous. I know I would be if I were in his shoes. I had no doubt that I will be cured! I love his concern and attention to detail to be prepared. I hoped he would see how tough I was throughout all this! I wanted him to feel comforted that this Speed Bump isn't huge, just a bump in our world. I kept thinking how I would have given anything to get cancer instead of losing Austin. His death was so debilitating for me. This isn't going to be that way! Nothing compares to losing my son.

I was anxious, not afraid, to get started on the battlefield against my cancer! Remember the Chemotherapy is a Treatment not a Tragedy! There is a learning curve with Chemotherapy for everyone. Listen to your body, it will help you to help yourself!

Going where my Body had Never been Before!
Chapter 4

First Chemotherapy Infusion

July 6th, almost a month from learning about the cancer Speed Bump. Amazing at how fast all the steps moved once we got the ball rolling. Walking into the infusion room the first thing I noticed, very inviting comfortable chairs.

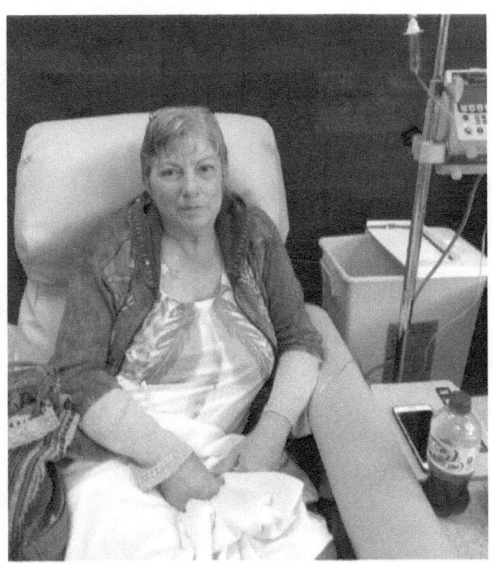

I know this is not a flattering picture but, getting infusions is not a beauty pageant. You need to be comfortable. The start of my new job of giving cancer hell!

The first Infusion starts as a slow injection of medications into the port. You will notice some patients will have a normal IV and others will have a port. The staff made me feel welcome and explained every step as it happened. My protocol called for seven IV bags of assorted sizes.

1. Dexamethasone
2. Diphenhydramine Hydrochloride (Benadryl®)
3. Famotidine
4. Pertuzumab
5. Trastuzumab (Herceptin®)
6. Taxotere
7. Paraplatin

Once they plugged the IV into my port the infusion began. My trusty backpack filled with snacks, peppermints, extra drink and tablet to check email, read or just surf the internet. I strongly suggest bringing supplies for time in the chair. Don't wear perfume or bring anything with a strong odor with your food. There are patients that may have nausea. I never had it and some of the medications they gave me I am sure prevented nausea.

The first infusion takes longer because they are slowly introducing it to your body to watch for any reactions. They take very seriously watching for reactions. I saw one person react with itching and a light rash. They stopped the infusion, gave her a shot, checked her pulse and blood pressure. Once she felt better, about ten minutes later, they started the infusion again. The woman didn't react again. The chairs make it very easy to take a nap! The only side effect I had at that infusion were leg aches caused by the Benadryl medication in one of the bags. The nurses said it was ok for me to take ibuprofen for the leg aches. After that I brought ibuprofen that I took when the Benadryl® started to relieve the leg aches. Never had a problem with that again. It can get cold for the patient while getting an infusion, they provided blankets and a pillow for napping. After the infusion finished they put what Jimmy and I called the robot on my upper right arm. During strong chemotherapy the drug Neulasta® is given the next day. It is a drug that is a white blood cell booster to reduce the risk of infection during strong chemotherapy. Many people go to the doctor's office the next day to receive a shot. The robot or technically called the On-body injector delivers the medication twenty-seven hours after it is placed on the body. When it is applied it is with an adhesive to the arm which automatically injects the catheter. Twenty-seven hours later it injects over about forty-five minutes the medication. Afterwards when it is finished it easily pulls off and is thrown away. I think the reason they used the robot instead of the shot the next day is that I qualified because we traveled 80 miles to the doctor's office. The first time of infusion is generally the longest because of the slow admission of the different drugs and monitoring. My first infusion took almost eight hours. The first time is a long day, but time well spent to get to the finish line!

The schedule is infusion, one week later a blood test and an appointment with the oncologist, then two weeks later is the next infusion. This schedule is throughout the chemotherapy infusions.

The following week they took blood to do the white count test and gather other information, followed by the appointment with my oncologist. This test and appointment are to check your blood counts, especially the white count and to touch base with the oncologist. The Doctor's main concern is the results of what you cannot see, the blood tests. They also like seeing the patient. If you have any questions at all or about your side effects that is when to would ask. Most of the time I didn't really have any questions. If you are having severe side effects before the appointment do not hesitate to call the Doctor. Jimmy and I just wanted to know my white cell count did not go down. That could delay treatment which would prolong getting them done. When I caught mono, my white count fell so low that it required the hospitalization. Then I was young and healthy! We took all precautions to keep me healthy and keep that white count good. Getting through the chemotherapy treatments is Priority One!

Jimmy had created the bubble for me. He also started enhancing the view out my window by adding a bird feeder and a bird bath so that I could see the birds come in for food and water.

It helped immensely to have him see everything going on from his point of view. Throughout he had some great suggestions and ideas. Jimmy had a wonderful suggestion when I started on day one of the chemotherapy treatment; keep a daily log of the side effects and how they felt. That is the best thing for any patient to do! The log gives you something to focus on and gives you control during the Chemo Fog. There will be days that there isn't much to write and others where you have several side effects. This log will help more for the following treatments, it gives you a sense of when a side effect may come on. Keep the log for each infusion day one to

day twenty-one, then do it again for the second treatment and on and
on.

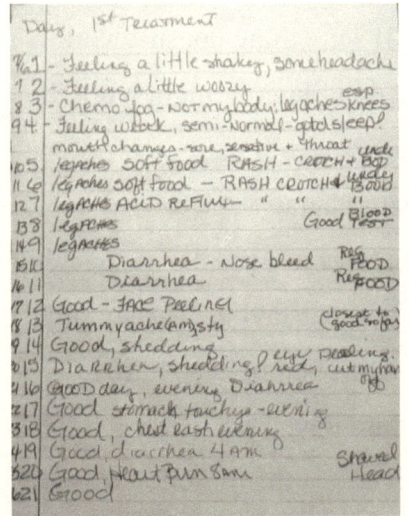 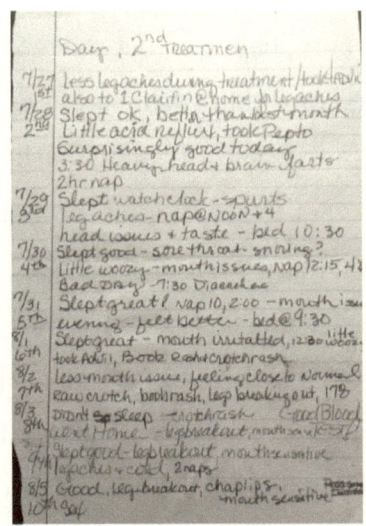

*Here are pictures of my log of the twenty-one days after my first and
second infusions. It is not pretty nor too organized, but worth its
weight in gold! Patterns start to appear.*

Most of the initial side effects were just plain weird. I kept
telling Jimmy in the beginning, "This does not feel like my body!"
Jimmy would look at me and say, "Yes, it is your body, luscious as
usual!" Then I would look in the mirror and realize I still looked the
same. Mostly I felt the Chemo Wave crashing on my brain synapses!

Days 1 -7 started with a general over all feeling of disconnect
with my body, leg aches and feeling weak. The rash in my crotch
area and under my boobs came next. The vitamin A & D® ointment
worked wonders for the crotch. Another immense help is wearing
loose underwear. As expected, I didn't have any loose underwear so
I asked Jimmy for suggestions. The brilliant man he is he went to the

bedroom and came back with a couple of pairs of his underwear! Perfect! Later I dyed some purple. Got to have style even wearing my husband's underwear! The rash under the boobs seemed more like a burn, baby powder relieved that. If something doesn't work the first time don't write it off, as I found out later it might work the next time. Especially on the rashes.

For two days after receiving chemotherapy you are toxic. No kissing, (hard habit to break) no sharing food or utensils, no touching while sleeping and no sex, which goes without saying. The sweat and other fluids from the body contains the chemotherapy drugs. That also pertains to sex, not until the third day. This for the protection of your spouse and/or caregiver. On the third day we washed the sheets and my clothes separate.

Next mouth changes. It became sore and sensitive. Soft food seemed best, mostly mashed potatoes. I am a flavor junkie when it comes to food! If mashed potatoes became my main food I wanted it loaded with sour cream, cheese and real butter! During that time, I didn't worry about calories, food needed to taste good! I also had a little bit of acid reflux too.

On day ten I went to the restroom and upon returning walking down the hall I rose my hands high and shouted, "Let the diarrhea begin!" Jimmy wanted to know how and what I felt each day, so I thought this one should be shouted to the roof tops! There is one pet peeve I have about talking about side effects, that certain one everybody whispers. We all know that it is one of the possible things with chemotherapy, yet the whisper mode kicks in with the

---

word diarrhea. It is one of those funny things that if we were talking about my grandson no one would go into whisper mode. Let it be an adult and the quieter diarrhea would be said. Little did I know that diarrhea would be around during most of the chemotherapy.

By day fourteen some face peeling, occasional diarrhea and unhappy digestion seemed to be effects at the time.

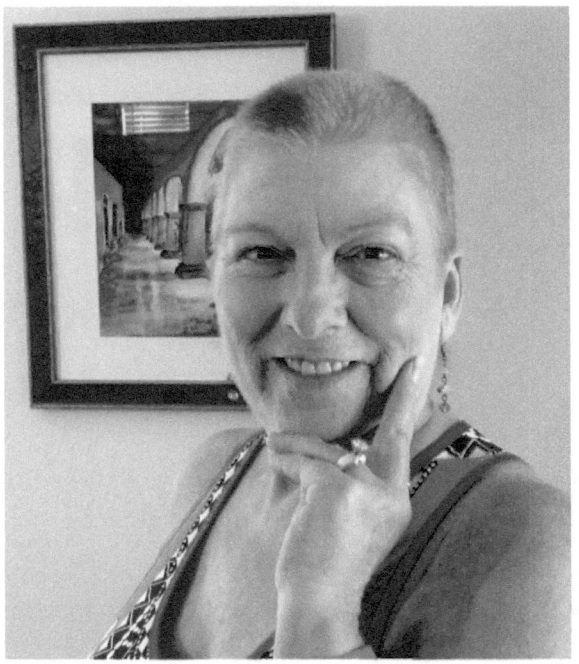

My Burr haircut!

As is predicted for most chemotherapy my hair started shedding on the twentieth day. When your pixie hair cut is coming out with every touch it seemed senseless to not move on to the next step. I told Jimmy that the time had come for hair shortening…a burr! The shedding had become an irritation landing on everything. Reminded me of Hansel and Gretel leaving bread crumbs all over the house. You could tell where I had been and where I hadn't been.

When it landed on my plate I declared it to be the last straw! Jimmy got out his electric hair shears and shaved my head for me!

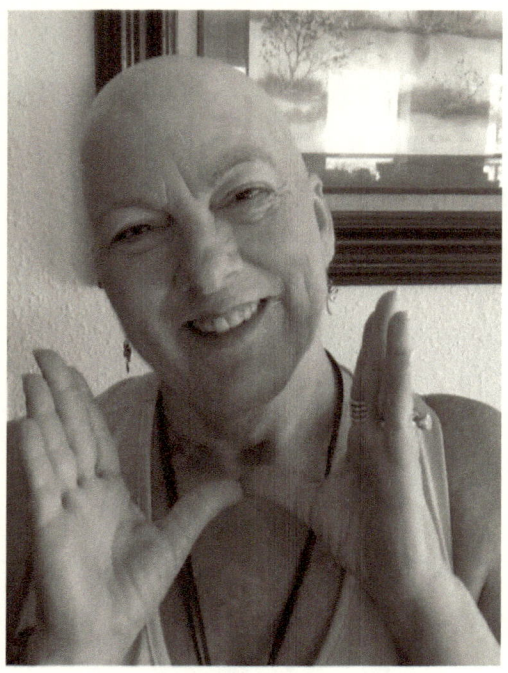

Yes, being bald is weird! When you first look in the mirror it does not sink in. Amazing how after a couple of days it felt normal.

What a relief for me. I know these last steps happened in a matter of days, but those steps helped me with the transition, whether it made sense or not. Letting it drag on would have been harder than not needing a brush!

I think that being bald helped with the hot and or heavy head, the wet paper towel on a bald head helps immediately! Sharing the disappearance of my hair on Facebook felt good to let everyone see, hoping that I can inspire others in some way. Especially if it helps them to encourage others to talk about it or feel free to contact me if they wish.

I must tell you, I had never thought about make-up issues after losing my hair. Talk about an interesting awakening! For one, where do you stop the base? No hair line, a bit of white area where the hair had been. Also, later the 'no eyebrows' are perplexing as that is a major part of expression. Where to stop eye shadow with no eyebrows? Not one woman had ever mentioned these issues. Then the realization that there were not any eyelashes. The monotone face, not my style. I am not big into make-up. I have always kept my make-up simple. Now I had a challenge. The normal routine for putting on my face really changed to putting on My Face! Your face becomes a blank palette. Thinking that way helped me to not worry about make-up lines. Buying an eyebrow pencil helped me put definition for expression, never had used one so you can image the experimental trials at first. I had thought about doing assorted color eyebrows for fun! Green eyebrows would make my expression noticeable. Grandchildren would laugh. In the end I just tried to make enough eyebrow look to have expression. My recommendation is to not stop wearing make-up. It may have some challenges but take those challenges with fun. I wore many assorted colors of eye shadow and added colored eyeliner. Remember when you were younger playing with make-up! Borrow or buy fun make-up! Experiment but do not stop using make-up! If it is part of making you feel feminine, Keep Doing It!

Having the Flu would be Worse
Chapter 5

Second of Six Chemotherapy Infusions

After this infusion 33% done! The Speed Bump of Boob Cancer was smaller! Jimmy and I found it amazing that before chemotherapy I could feel my lump easily as it was just under the skin. Now I literally could not feel the lump easily! One other thing we found helpful is that while I was getting my infusion Jimmy would run errands. This gives the caregiver time to do things that may be time consuming. This provided an easy way for Jimmy to get things accomplished knowing that I had someone taking care of me.

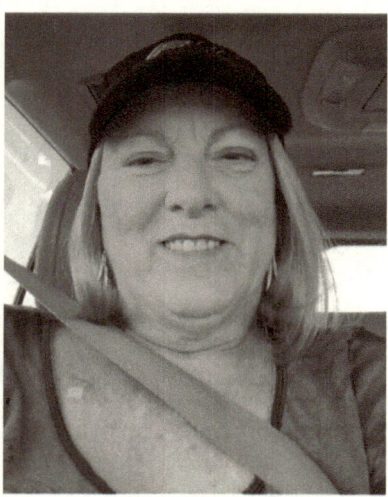

On the way to number two of six. Knowing that I had made it through the first one!

Raising four kids I hardly ever got sick, so going through Chemotherapy I expected from day-one to crash. That did not happen. The first five days were the hardest. The leg aches seemed much less, the Chemo Wave caused the brain farts to kick in. My head felt heavy and hot. A wet paper towel may have looked funny on my head, but it sure did feel fantastic! I didn't wear hats or wigs very often, mostly to go to the doctor and infusions. It was a comfortable change from hair down to my butt to a bald beauty. I did use shampoo when showering, what can I say, I love the smell of my shampoo!

A weather event happened that we did not expect. The arrival of a heat wave! Then, with perfect timing, our central air conditioning went out! The central air unit had been around a long time, so I can't say we were surprised but the timing had to be now? Jimmy knew the probability of it being on its last leg so to be prepared he ordered window units. He is always ready with a backup and backup to that backup! We had this happen years ago when we lived here before and found that the window units did an excellent job. The heat became my enemy and my loving caregiver made sure I did not feel uncomfortable for a minute. He even put an extra window unit in the window across the room that pointed straight in my direction. Walking outside felt like hitting a wall of heat and made it difficult to make it to the car.

I napped each day, partially because I could not sleep very well at night. The naps seem to help with the heavy head, but not the brain farts! Most of the side effects returned after this infusion almost to the day of the last twenty-one-day cycle. Keeping the log is what helps in knowing when to expect things that may reappear or not show at all. Many of the side effects come and go. The raw mouth and tongue became the most frustrating. At one point, the texture of bread in my mouth was torture to eat. The taste buds were changing almost daily. The day that my mouth didn't like chocolate shocked me! My wonderful husband makes me Boyfriend Coffee every morning that includes chocolate, he couldn't believe he had to skip the chocolate. Another bizarre change my taste buds pulled took place when my normal artificial sweetener brand tasted terrible, so we changed to another brand for a short time. Then that changed to it had to be sugar. Not regular sugar, it had to be brown sugar! Making a list of foods you miss is an excellent way to reward yourself when eating normal is possible on the second half of the three-week cycle. Part of the caregiver's job is to keep the patient eating. Jimmy took that very seriously! He bought a fryer to fix my favorite foods. It became his secret weapon. He fixed me a huge seafood platter with fried fish, fried shrimp and potato wedges when my mouth returned to normal! He excelled at being a very attentive caregiver! Remember to thank your caregiver, they are doing everything they can to help you.

An odd side effect that popped up on day seven, my left leg broke out. They started as either a pus pocket or a knot under the skin the size of a marble. Some were sore to the touch, others became what we called boils when I was a kid. The strange thing is that it mostly broke out on the left side of my body, predominately the left leg. My face and torso looked like getting a mild case of acne. The alternating of hydrocortisone, triple antibiotic and airing out the boils worked best, this lasted generally about a week.

The diarrhea arrived right on time! My log is filled with misspells of diarrhea with the Chemo Fog. Little did I understand it would return every cycle like a boomerang! Anti-diarrhea medicine became my best friend. The digestive system side effects are due to how the chemotherapy can damage the healthy cells of the lining of the whole digestive system, including the mouth. All the linings are affected which leads to issues you may have to deal with. Nausea never cropped up as a problem for me. As I said before, part of the drugs of infusion are to help with nausea and irritation of the digestive system. My understanding is that they have made great strides keeping the nausea under control for chemotherapy patients.

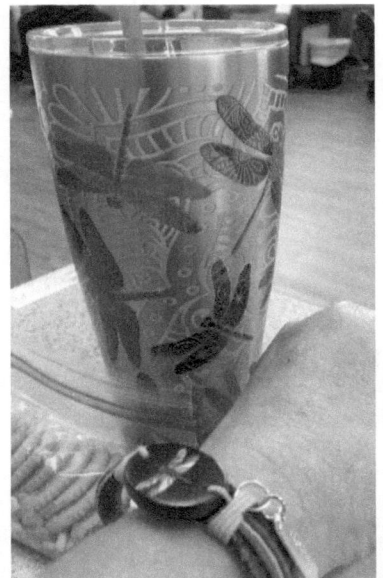

A wonderful surprise came in the mail! Lynn sent me a bracelet with a dragonfly and the word "Hope." They also sent a dragonfly glass and Carter sent an Angel metal disk to carry. I was very touched. I love dragonflies!

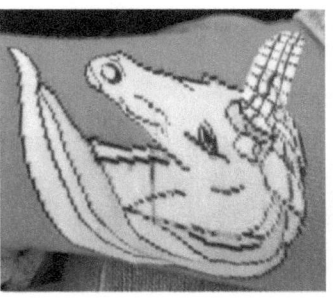

During the rest of my treatments I carried that glass everywhere I went. My grandson Spencer had given me lucky Unicorn socks too. I carried and wore all the gifts of love!

On the eleventh day I could see and feel the sunshine of "normal" peeking out. Bloating and restless sleep were what I had to deal with for a couple of days. Lemon tea helped with the bloating and eased my stomach. Also added probiotic yogurt to my daily routine to help give the digestive system what it needed to return to normal.

At this point Jimmy added a Rainbow Garden Spinner and Sail! The vibrant colors popped and when the wind blew the three wheels spun. It took a day for the animals to get comfortable with it being out there. Jimmy also moved the shooting bench where I could see him out the window when he could do some target shooting. Two days later we woke up to see the cows had gotten over the cattle guard and destroyed everything Jimmy had done in the garden! We were shocked that they did all that destruction for a couple of cups of bird seed! Phoebe even helped by chasing a two-thousand-pound bull out of the yard! She grew up as a puppy with our white German Shepherd, guess she still doesn't realize how little she is. I laughed to see the bull scared of her! Jimmy decided the time had come to fix the cattle guard with the tractor. Unfortunately, he broke the hydraulic hoses while mowing and moving dead trees into a pile. He made an enormous attempt to fix it, but the limitation of tools hindered his getting it done. We knew the tractor hadn't had the normal maintenance in a very long time, so we decided it needed go into the shop. Delay for the cattle guard repair. This began the declaration proclaimed loudly of us saying "We hate these cows!" These cows were not ours. A neighbor was leasing to keep his cows there. When we had cattle, they had manners! Hence the irritation of ill-mannered cows!

By the sixteenth day I thoroughly enjoyed feeling quite normal. We were thrilled to have some time that was not consumed by the side effects before the third chemotherapy session. Being able to eat normally and the fatigue to go away encouraged me to conquer the next treatment!

Jimmy told me that he had begun planning on getting the pop-up ready so that when we were all done we can go on a camping trip to celebrate "Living." We would go back to our favorite spot in Big Bend under the stars, back to our reason to live there and ground with nature and the beauty created. His talking of the future gave me the encouragement I needed to hear and is good for anyone going through chemotherapy.

Slammed by a Sneaky
Consuming Side Effect
Chapter 6

Third of Six Chemotherapy Infusions

Don't let the side effects scare you, they had been manageable. My white blood count continued to be at the top of normal. Jimmy created the bubble for me and took every step to make it enjoyable and comfortable while being away from home during my treatments. My bubble was at the family ranch that is seventeen miles from town. It is in central Texas, very wooded and down a dirt road. Our friends would tease us when we lived there that we were in the witness protection program! We would send them directions but most of the time we had to talk them in or meet them at a main road. When Jimmy went to get groceries or the pharmacy I didn't go into stores unless absolutely necessary, which ended up being twice during all six treatments. I enjoyed being able to see my kids and grandchildren occasionally when the time was good for me and no one had any sickness. At this time, I started really sharing everything about this experience with family and friends on social media. I was felt it was important that I share the details of the side effects with everyone. If anything, I wanted to share because hardly anyone talks about what they go through with cancer. It provided an avenue to offer information and help to anyone that wanted to ask questions.

I walked into the Doctors office excited to be there! August 17th getting the third infusion and that meant I would be half way! Woohoo! We also looked forward to seeing friends we had made who have the same schedule and the staff. The relationships had developed with the wonderful staff at Austin Cancer Center. The treatment time diminished down to four and one-half hours! It was still enough time for visiting, a nap and to check email.

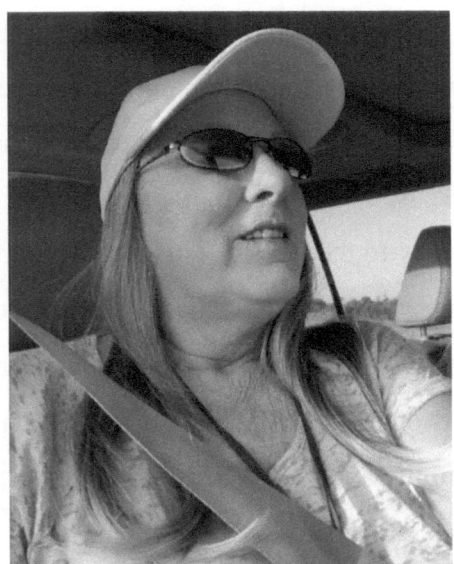

On the way to the third infusion wearing the hat with attached wig. I ended up using this one most of the time

Starting on day three after my infusion the acid reflux, diarrhea and wooziness came on fast and furious. Woozy for me is the room spinning. Dizzy is me spinning! I am accustomed to fainting from having a history of fainting all my life and have developed the tools to stop it before it happens. My kids grew up knowing when mom said, "I am going down," they would get a cold wet cloth to hand me. It didn't happen often but the time I hit my elbow on the microwave, I announced "I am going down!" Suddenly I had a cold wet wash cloth and a cold wet bath towel! Don't know if the bath towel was clean, as the utility is located next the microwave. The quick reaction is what counted!

Diarrhea gave me fits. I spent a majority of the first week, eating, drinking and sleeping. The problems of the digestive system are also the inability to absorb fluids. The linings of the stomach, digestive system throughout your body basically are destroyed. Those days I spent napping too much, not drinking enough and lost nine pounds. On the seventh day we went to the appointment for my blood count check. At that point I had tremendous trouble staying conscious on the way to the doctor. This wasn't fainting, this was something I am unaccustomed to. Still we carried a cold wet cloth on my head to help as we drove to the appointment with my oncologist. I kept losing consciousness off and on during the drive. As you may guess, it scared Jimmy and me! When we walked in, the doctor looked at me, pinched the skin on my arm and said, "You are dehydrated." The relief of hearing that was incredible! Thank goodness, something manageable, not a blood count problem. Straight into the infusion room I went. The staff there knew I felt terrible, I never go in without an enthusiastic greeting. They plugged into my port and started an IV with a large bag of saline solution. In twenty minutes, I babbled like usual and felt like a whole new person! In hind sight we should have called and gone in a day or two earlier.

When we returned home I declared this would Not happen again! We also learned that because the diarrhea is problematic it is better to stock up with a bigger quantity of the anti-diarrhea medication. Jimmy found a generic brand that came in larger quantities and didn't cost a fortune. The research I did gave me the answers to keep hydrated. I love mathematics, give me the equation and I will take it and run! Got this figured out!

3 Quarts of fluids a Day = keeping hydrated and human! I have never been a big water drinker to say the least. Daily fluids for me before cancer included caffeinated coffee and soda. The important part of fluids I learned, Not Just Water! Pinching my skin became part of the daily routine at least twice a day. Electrolyte solution (for babies) or sports drink proved to be a huge help! Bouillon is suggested but didn't work for me. Jimmy pulled the seasoning packets out of ramen noodles which worked miracles to help my body to retain the fluids. Thank goodness Jimmy thinks outside the box! Monitoring hydration is a strong suggestion I would make for anyone going into Chemotherapy. There are other benefits that accompany keeping hydrated during the treatments such as flushing your system after the infusions to help get the toxins out of your body those first couple of days after each infusion.

There will be things such as weather for us along the Gulf of Mexico that may throw an event into your plans. Jimmy and I have grown up with hurricanes all our lives. When one starts, we take notice, no matter how far out it is. The hurricane season of 2017 being extremely active kept our attention to each storm as it moved to see if any of them needed to be watched closely. That is the one thing I have always been thankful for about hurricanes, you do have some time to prepare if it possibly is headed your way. Everyone that has lived in hurricane area keeps the standard base of equipment or should keep supplies to be ready with a little time to prepare. We have always, even as a kid known to be prepared. Growing up we were one of the first families on our block to have a generator, that was a huge help! Now, that is standard along with flashlights, charcoal, lighter fluid, propane, water containers, dry goods, canned goods and on and on. Jimmy has always been ready for a hurricane and always had a backup to the backup! I have never had to worry about an emergency. It is a running joke that Jimmy has plan A, B, C, D and E! Jimmy checked all the supplies, went to get extra gas and can goods. At this point it looked like hurricane Harvey aimed at hitting the Texas gulf coast. While at our visit with my doctor we talked with him about whether to stay at the ranch or go home to Alpine. We have huge issues with flooding at the ranch. When it floods you cannot get out and it can last for weeks. Our biggest concern, dehydration. If it happened again and I would need the saline solution. Even with all the preparation for the hurricane we made the decision we would go home. Westward Ho we went! Jimmy worried more about getting the saline solution if needed and my reaction to heat. Loss of electricity would mean no air conditioning and there would be the slam of weakness and fainting. Of course, while at home we watched the devastating effects of

Hurricane Harvey. We had family in the path of destruction and torrential down pours of rain. Thank goodness no one was hurt. Everyone had damage and loss, but things can be replaced. I could not stop thinking about the other patients that couldn't get in for their infusions.

While back in Alpine for that week, it made Jimmy very uncomfortable about not being able to protect and take care of me as easily. The Bubble Jimmy created was where I felt most comfortable and safe from germs. It was also so much easier for Jimmy.

When we returned to the ranch our first sight was the total destruction of the garden! We both exclaimed "We hate these cows!" Jimmy is not daunted easily! He added two deer feeders for me to be able to see deer. The deer found the feeders within two days! Jimmy and I talked about planting oats too as soon as the tractor came back!

After the third infusion the side effects included; rash in the crotch and under the boobs, bloated stomach, gas, sores with knots on my leg and sore mouth. All lessened as I reached the fifteenth day after treatment, except the diarrhea. The diarrhea being one of the serious issues that contributed to the dehydration I tried to drink the necessary fluids. Eating became a problem, I began eating noodles and puddings to try to keep something in my stomach at least six to eight times a day. I felt good enough for sex the last seven days before the next infusion. You may not feel pretty. Do what makes you feel cute. Remember this look is temporary! We have always had a healthy sex life. The interference of the raw feeling in the vagina makes it painful. I was determined to not give up sex. My body and I love the endorphins and adrenalin from sex. It is important to not delete the closeness with your lover. They need the closeness as much or more than you while battling cancer. Remember they are watching you, sometimes feeling helpless. Keep that connection strong with sex when you can, but also remember that talking is another form of intercourse.

At this point in my treatment a nap every day was necessary. The naps were part of our routine. It did give Jimmy time to do a few things that he needed to do and not be distracted with watching me.

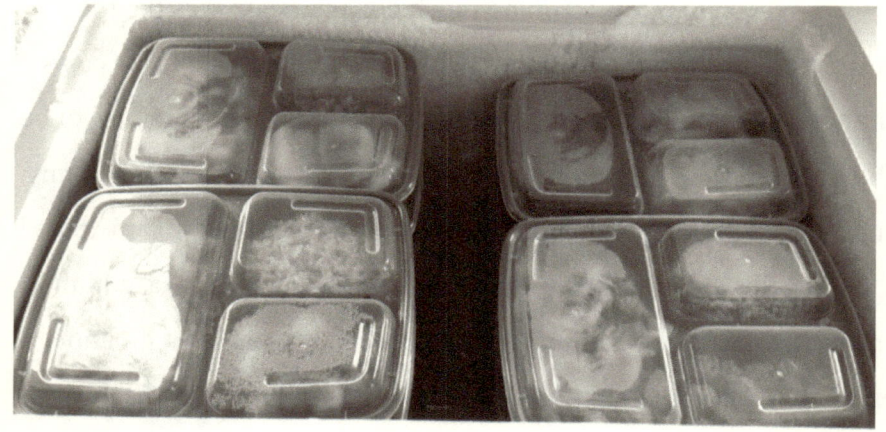

Since Jimmy did not need to cook for two he made up frozen dinners for him. I thought, what a brilliant idea!

Up to this point I had been trying to do as much as I could. Dishes and laundry are the areas that I don't like anyone else to do! I have my routine and patience for both. That had gone out the window at this point in my treatment! Poor Jimmy had to take over those chores also on top of everything else. I guess my biggest pet peeve at this point, bed making. It is one of those things I do every day! Call me obsessed, but I like crawling into a made bed at night. Due to the fatigue and napping I could not make the bed every morning, much less keep it made with the naps. Like many of the other trivial things, I gave myself a break. I must tell you that now I especially enjoy climbing into a made bed more that I used to!

Twinkle at the End
of the Chemotherapy Tunnel
Chapter 7

Fourth of Six Chemotherapy Infusions

Knowing that this infusion began the second half gave me the boost to feel energized for the downhill side of treatments. The end of the tunnel has a light like the North Star. Now all I had to do, follow it!

At this point my brain fell into full Chemo Fog! Many days the best part consisted of sitting around in one of Jimmy's button-up shirts and his underwear. I felt so comfortable and it helped to be relaxed while handling side effects. The simpler my day the easier for me.

The infusion time was faster this time. As you progress and have no signs of reaction they can speed up the drip. Even with my snacks I always came out starving afterwards! Jimmy would run get something for when I got out to eat. My side effects after this infusion included rash, (*loose clothing helped loads*) acid reflux and diarrhea in the beginning. Adding probiotic yogurt again to my routine helped my digestion. Again, the irritating bloating and burping. Little did I realize that the burping would return routinely with every treatment. Remember I told you to ask question about side effects at the appointment. I would suggest using some common sense...they probably can't do anything about burping! I have always as a mother and grandmother corrected the kids to say, "Excuse me." Now I had uncontrollable burping! Talk about embarrassing! I could be in mid-sentence and suddenly explode an enormously loud burp. For Jimmy and me it became hilarious at how inconvenient and comical with the many times my body would erupt! My grandson heard me burp and turned to me, "Gammaw! Did you do that?" The look of shock on his face was priceless.

The leg break-out of knots and a boil happened again after this treatment. Coupled with leg aches, my legs were a bit of a pain this time. Ibuprofen helped with the leg aches. Keeping the boil clean is a priority. Alternating with triple antibiotic ointment, hydrocortisone cream and leaving it uncovered every third day brought the best results to help it heal.

Some days I couldn't muster the energy for a shower, it exhausted me. We put a plastic chair in the shower and Jimmy stood there to help me get in and out. Weakness and dizziness became the major factor in showering. I had problems with closing my eyes to wash my face without losing my balance. Take precautions bathing and if you can't, just take a wash cloth bath. It won't hurt to skip a day, just keep any irritated areas clean.

There is the side effect I call Heavy Head. It was hard to describe to Jimmy. My best explanation is that my head felt like having a weighted hat on. Reminded me of walking around with a five-pound book on my head! Did not help my posture though!

The lotion for the skin is important. During the chemotherapy treatments I tried to remember to put it on. For me that wasn't as big of a problem as I have normally moist skin. Only during very dry chilly days during winter do I sometimes need lotion. For those who have dry or light skin, lotion may be part of your daily routine. The face peeling ended up happening every time. It would peel at least three times after each infusion. The peeling did not cause any pain but did cause some problems with putting on My Face. Definitely looked like I had been getting microdermabrasion sessions. One very surprising side effect, chapped lips popped up. Even though I had never used lip balm, it brought a wonderful relief.

Didn't have as strong of a problem with dehydration after this infusion. Partially because of the knowledge needed to understand how to help keep it under control. The three things that helped me the most to fight dehydration included water, electrolyte solution (for babies) and seasoning packets of ramen noodles. It reminded me of breaking the rules from when the kids were growing up. I constantly fussed at my kids for taking the seasoning packets out. Back then I would get a ramen package out, boil the water, reach for the package to find it already open. Seasoning packet missing! Just one of those little things that was more frustrating when I was fixing it for them when they were sick. I had to share with my now grown kids that I had broken the rule of the ramen noodles for a hot cup of broth for dehydration. The best part is now we use broken ramen noodles for a salad topper!

Dizziness continued to be an issue. As I told my best friend Sharon, "It is hard being a dizzy blonde without my hair!" The dizziness seemed to be worse right after an infusion. There were times that I swear my head was emitting heat. Then there were other times my head felt like it had water sloshing around inside. Reminded me of a snow globe, with brain cells bouncing around after I moved my head! Really blew my mind when it happened, and I had not moved my head!

One of the funny parts is that other side effects from earlier treatments had diminished or stopped! No one ever mentioned that! The only annoying side effect that has been since day one, were odd and sensitive taste buds and mouth. Poor Jimmy had to deal with it changing day to day! Imagine having to cook for erratic, picky, schizophrenic taste buds! Much less grocery shopping! My quest for flavor that didn't hurt when I ate became challenging and sometimes expensive. My recommendation is to keep trying, but, don't buy too much of any one thing. Sour cream lasted for five days and then it stung my tongue. Treat yourself to food that might normally be a treat, especially if you are trying not to lose weight. I tried to keep my weight the same by adding the extras. Due to dehydration and the pesky mouth issue, I would drop ten pounds and my skin looked ten years older. By the next infusion I gained back the loss to get back to my normal weight. This is important as they measure the drugs by your weight and losing weight can cause other issues that you don't need while on chemotherapy.

Going through chemotherapy is not a walk in the park. Most

of the time after my fourth treatment I felt just like when I had mononucleosis as a teenager. I had a couple of days that pushed back on me. Then Jimmy would say just what encouragement I needed. One day I said, "Thank you, I needed that!" He responded, "That's what a caretaker does." I broke out in laughter! "You mean caregiver, not caretaker!" We both giggled about that the rest of the day. Proves love and laughter are the best medicine!

I can see there is a Finish Line
Chapter 8

Fifth of Six Infusions

It still amazed me how some of the side effects had disappeared. Not bad, just not what I expected. I thought it was going to be horrid after this infusion! Unfortunately for Jimmy my taste buds were still getting sore and picky! Pepper became the enemy for my mouth! I started collecting recipes to cook after chemotherapy. My sister, Lynne, is the chef out of the two of us. So many times, I laughed that she would hunt out old recipe books when we went out together browsing around. Now I began looking for the recipes from our childhood. I had a strong desire for those flavors of old-fashioned dishes. Also looked for ways to cook favorite vegetables that enhanced their delicious uniqueness. Most of the hunger for specific taste had to be the result of having to eat bland food and most food didn't taste like normal. Jimmy helped me to find foods that tasted good to keep my interest in eating. We learned to be creative with foods, sauces and condiments. Ketchup became the foe, but honey mustard dressing was heavenly! All my normal favorites in the beginning, like ranch dressing, sour cream, cream cheese and butter, that helped me in the beginning of chemotherapy now tasted terrible! I love butter on almost anything, normally. I never ever thought butter could taste offensive!

Two new side effects appeared, vision and hearing, it proved to be shall we say interesting? My vision changed so much that my prescription seemed very inadequate. I had to buy stronger reading glasses to wear with my contacts to compensate. Easy fix for the problem though.

My hearing created a whole other issue! Poor Jimmy had to deal with picky taste buds AND my unstable hearing! Everyday my hearing could be amplified, diminished, reverberating, ringing or nonexistent. Some days Jimmy had to repeat himself so often it had to be exhausting. Other days I would have to ask him to use his "Inside Voice". We found the best solution, I kept charge of the volume control for the television. It gave him a hint as to how my hearing seem to be doing each day! I found many ways to ask people to repeat themselves. One time at infusion while talking with some friends and their family, one of the brothers asked me a question and I literally did not understand a word out of his mouth. The other brother looked at me when I didn't respond. I asked him to repeat what he had asked. On the second time I still could not hear what he said. I looked at both brothers and told them I was sorry I cannot hear either of them. Thank goodness Jimmy turned around to answer the question. The ultimate feeling of frustration! They were both very kind and understanding.

An odd thing happened after the fifth treatment. We went home for a short visit. Our home is in the mountains with the altitude at just under 5,000 feet. At the ranch it is at about 500 feet in altitude. I have vertigo at 10,000+ feet normally. After arriving home, I started just feeling a bit worse than before. By the time we had been there, about forty-eight hours it became obvious that I was experiencing vertigo. The best we could figure happened is because of hair loss everywhere. In addition to hair loss on your legs, arm pits, arms, crotch, face, head and even your toes, there is hair loss in your nose and the sensory hairs in the inner ears. Who would have thought hair loss would kick off my vertigo? By the time we went home again, it was after surgery and my hair had started growing again. I never thought I would be glad to see nose hairs growing. The sign I used to assume that my ear sensory hairs had grown too.

The rash returned like an explosion. It felt more like a burn from the toxicity of sweating. The baby powder didn't help. Jimmy suggested putting his deodorant under my boobs. That was the ticket! The irritation stopped and soothed the rash. The sore lumps and boils began on time. There seemed to be less of the sore bumps, but the boil came back the same size and took the same amount of time to diminish following the same routine for it.

Burping can be very irritating! My word, I didn't think my body could burp that often or that much. In the month I believe I burped a life time's worth! The one good thing about not going into public, not having to worry about embarrassing myself or Jimmy with my constant burping. We marked it up to be the one funny side effect obviously opposite of my normal.

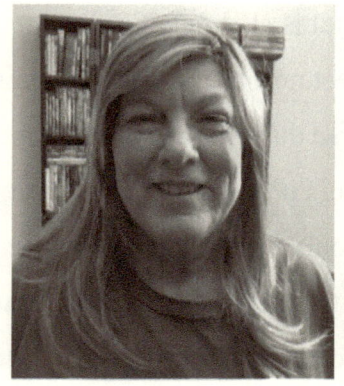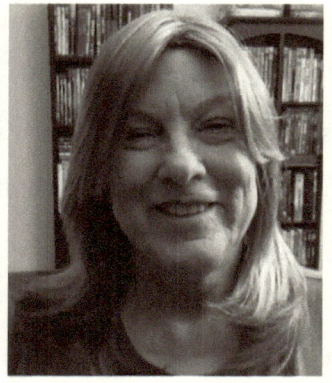

At this point I tried the wig thing. Surprisingly they are less expensive than I thought so we bought four for me to try....

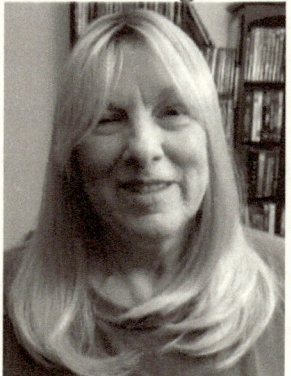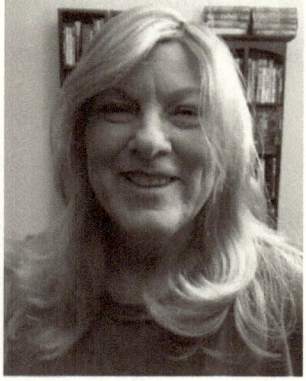

It did not prove to be as much fun as I had imagined as a kid! I ended up using one of them sometimes. After finishing all my treatments, I donated them to the drama department at Sul Ross University in Alpine.

There were a couple of days that I had a sore throat which happens with mouth issues for many people. The headaches came on about the same time, but continued off and on, the whole three weeks. The trusty side effect of diarrhea came on, right on time. The best part of keeping a daily log of what you are feeling, it gives timing of side effects that are repetitive.

Occasionally I had trouble with sleeping at night. It did not seem to matter if I had taken a nap that day or not. Some of the sleeplessness was due to feeling uncomfortable and at other times just being awake. In fact, one night I woke up at 3 AM. That night I kept thinking about how some friends suggested I write a book about my breast cancer experience. This had stemmed from the Facebook posts I had been doing after every treatment. Talking about the breast cancer experience would help people have knowledge and understanding. Since I could not sleep, I grabbed paper and pen, started writing. I knew that I wanted to write a book that would have helped me after finding out I had HER2-positive Boob Cancer. That night I began the process of putting everything into words as if talking to my best friend or a family member.

Finally, we got the tractor back! Yes! First thing Jimmy did, pull the cattle guard and reset it, so the cows could not come in again! Thank goodness! They created entertainment watching them try to get in! A puzzle they never would figure out. Jimmy also planted oats in the area by the deer feeders. This would be a big help for the deer.

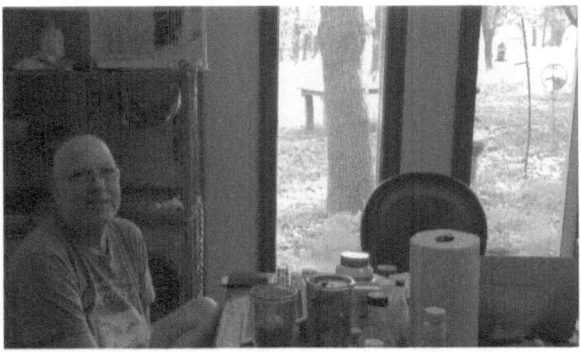

These three weeks turned out to be a bit harder. Here is a picture of me just sitting in my bubble by my window at the ranch.

The fatigue and weakness had become cumulative for me. The good part, the cumulative effects only became obvious after my fifth treatment! Naps became part of my daily routine the whole time. Just folding clothes, I would run out of energy as my arms grew very weak. From the beginning of my chemotherapy I had been trying to do as much as possible of my normal routine of washing and folding clothes as I said earlier. By this treatment, those types of tasks were absolutely impossible. At this point I kept thinking how difficult it must be for other patients who had work and raising a family. I was so thankful that this had happened in a time in our life that we could take a year to handle it. Considering it being the next to last treatment I didn't let it get me down, I felt like I had the flu plus. One time I had the flu, one of the very rare times I got sick while raising my children. Of course, back then I had an endless task list, but I remember the frustration of not being able to muster energy to do anything. Back then it lasted for only a few days. Thank goodness, laundry adds up quick with a family of six!

Ring That Bell!
Chapter 9

Last of Six Chemotherapy Infusions

There were three days until my last chemotherapy treatment. Jimmy and I had spent the day relaxing and reflecting on being so close to finishing with the chemotherapy step of our cancer Speed Bump. We had finished an early dinner when Jimmy's phone rang. He answered it starting to talk to our son-in-law Rob, Amy's husband. It seems that Amy had fallen thru the floor of their attic about twelve feet and had broken her leg. Rob assured us that she was ok. The ambulance had left to take her to the hospital. Our grandson at that time was about eighteen months old and Rob needed us to meet him at the hospital to get Kain to take care of him. It is funny how fast a parent can move when their child is hurt at three or thirty. On the drive to Kyle we wondered about the extent of her injury, hoping for just a cast. When we arrived, Rob stood outside with Kain. Jimmy had developed a wonderful close relationship with Kain, so he jumped to PaPaw. Rob took me into the ER to see Amy. It seems that she not only broke her leg but also her ankle. They were taking x-rays, so we had to wait at the door. I saw the pictures of the x-rays and knew it had many breaks. The look on my face when I walked in and saw her leg must have been one of shock. Her leg looked like a hockey stick!

Amy had been very aware of keeping my white count good. When I walked into her ER room she immediately started fussing at me about being there! As we all know if you are avoiding catching something, walking into an emergency room is the first on a list of no-no's! I had to see my child hence I did not even think about it. I talked with her for a very few minutes and gave her a hug. When we went back outside Rob held Kain and I took Jimmy inside to show him to Amy's room. She gave me That Look and told me to go back outside! I couldn't help but laugh that she was the one hurt and panicked that I could be getting exposed to germs by coming in the ER!

We took Kain home with us back to the ranch. Kain had been still breast feeding and had never stayed away from mommy! (*also, Kain had never had a bottle*) Amy said that he normally went to sleep around 2 A.M. Rob works till ten at night, so their schedule runs late. That did not match with our schedule, so Kain had to learn the first night to sleep with us and not mommy at ten. All the women in the family called Jimmy the next day to ask "Did Kain sleep last night?" I told Jimmy it happened to be perfect timing, being in my good week before chemotherapy. Rob took off from work to be there for Amy and to come help us with Kain. When Rob came out to stay with Kain he asked how we got him to bed because he had "never actually put him down." We giggled, and Jimmy told him "he needed to create his own style to put Kain to bed." Jimmy had his hands full taking care of me and Kain which exhausted Jimmy, but he never complained. He is such a trooper!

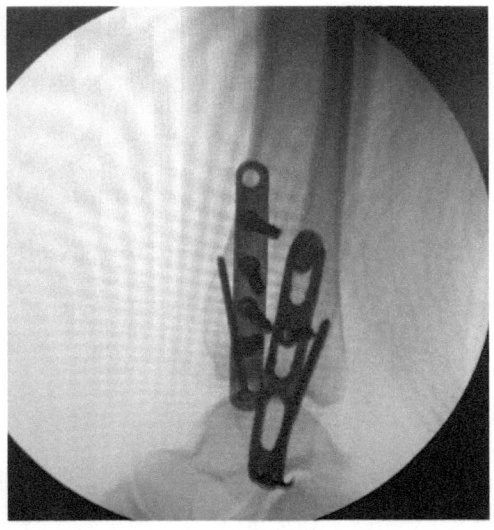

Amy had her operation which they put pins, plates and lots of stitches. Here is a picture of the x-ray after her surgery.

Jimmy pulled out the walker and shower chair we had gotten for Lynne. The wheelchair arrived and between it and the walker, Amy could maneuver around. They stayed with us for a couple days after Amy got out of the hospital then went home. We could not be more thankful that Rob's family came in to help while Amy recovered.

As I started my last infusion on October 19th, I remembered a woman I met on my first infusion. She had HER2-positive the same protocol as mine, except it was her last infusion. She's about 15 years older than myself and her husband is like Jimmy, with her always. Through my infusions I watched her, seeing the changes shine brightly in her. She looked so cute in her new wig, and energetic smile while walking hand in hand with her husband. We met many people that liked how we talk about issues and remedies for chemotherapy side effects. Along with Jimmy's ease to talk and lighten up the room, it seemed to help the other patients and families feel free to chat. In the end Cancer is Cancer, everyone feels like comrades, no matter the difference in their cancer or protocol.

The side effects of my final infusion could not have been predicted. For the first time the rash, burping, gas and acid reflux came on the day of treatment. Second day started with heavy head, dizziness and diarrhea. Diarrhea coming on so fast, we fought dehydration. Everything cumulative with a vengeance. Most of the time after each infusion it took 36 to 48 hours before most of the side effects started. This time, more like a hidden snake had jumped up and bit me. The chemo brain emerged in full effect, so it was very helpful at the follow-up for Jimmy to be able to tell the doctor what the side effects were. As I have said, they take the side effects seriously. It is helpful all during treatment to have your caregiver with you when you meet with your doctor. The chemo brain will hinder your ability to remember everything you are experiencing and any questions you may have.

On day three finger tips and nails felt numb, followed the next day with being sore. These were a first. Upon some research I discovered it to be a common side effect of the chemotherapy medication in my protocol. My toes joined the numb club a week later. The finger nails started to discolor and lift from the nail bed. The toe nails did not follow, but still had numb toes. The nail changes can be brittleness, yellowing, looking bruised under the nail and can lift off the nail bed as mine did. I had to start keeping them short to keep them from getting caught on something and pay more attention to keeping them dry under the nail. It's relatively easy by taking the edge of a torn paper towel and placing it in-between the nail and nail bed to keep it dry. Avoiding cleaners, harsh chemicals and water, for example; washing dishes, gloves are an immense help to keep from infection. After a shower or bath, checking to make sure the water is not under the nail is very important.

The numbness of the finger tips seemed much less than the toes. According to my research there are some chemotherapy drugs which can cause peripheral neuropathy. It is referred to as Chemotherapy-Induced Peripheral Neuropathy (CIPN). It is damage to nerves that control the sensations and movements of our arms and legs. There are other symptoms such as pain for CIPN that I did not have. For me just numbness of my toes at this point after my last infusion.

My nasal passages became very dry which caused nose bleeds. Blowing you nose is something you take for granted. Ha! It can be shocking to blow and then realize you just dyed the tissue or soft paper towel in my case. The three weeks after the last infusion the sides effects continued. Mostly the issues of digestion, diarrhea, hearing, heavy head, boils, weakness, mouth sensitivity and fatigue. By this time, I did not feel better physically, but mentally thrilled because it would be the last time to experience these side effects.

I was not sleeping well, and my taste buds were numb, but I ate a Sonic hamburger that I had been craving and enjoyed Sex!

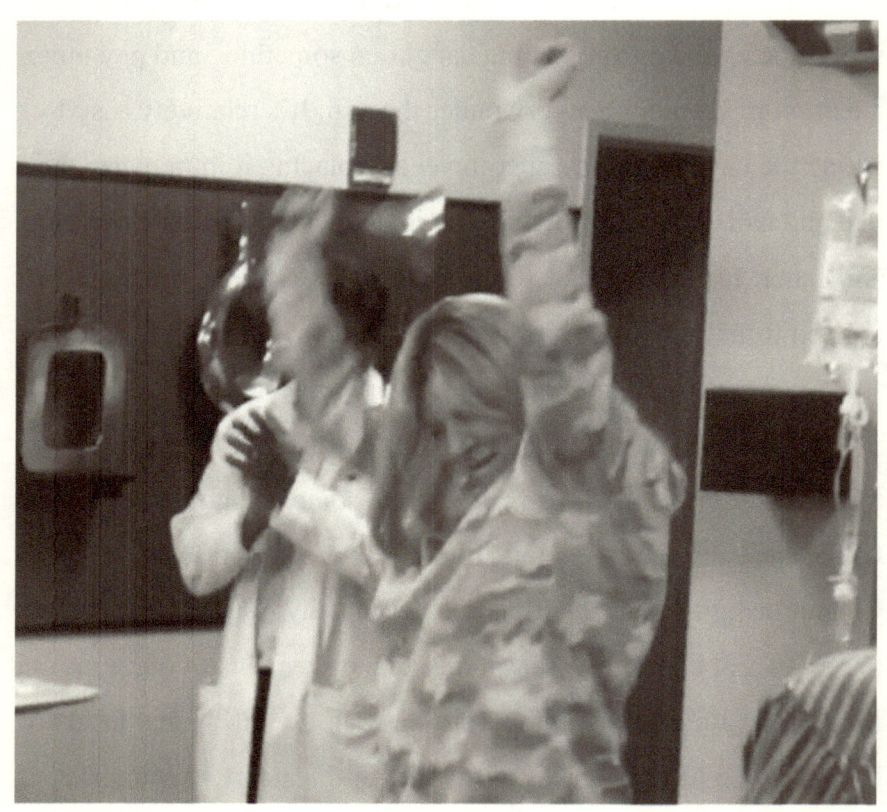

Ringing That Bell! A tradition of finishing Chemotherapy. This is a moment to be very proud of!

The support of those in the infusion room, the receptionist, the nurses and my doctors all came in to cheer me on to Ring the Bell! What a wonderful feeling of accomplishment and support from all that were a part of these steps in fighting Boob Cancer! My wonderful medical team was a huge part of the amazing encouragement needed when battling this unseen force.

We felt so excited about my final infusion. Chemotherapy Done! Jimmy had grown tired of watching me get poisoned. He said it was like watching them give me gasoline. Jimmy wanted to protect me, but he couldn't as the chemotherapy was important to kill the cancer.

It had been 5 ½ months since the phone rang. Chemotherapy had taken 4 ½ months. This is the hardest part because it is so time consuming and long. The passion to Ring the Bell is partially because the worst half is over and to feel the accomplishment of completing that big step of the protocol!

It would be thrilling to be the last time for side effects. I would be able to eat normally! On the way back to the ranch Jimmy asked me 'What would you like to celebrate your finishing?" I didn't have to think about it. I wanted Taco Bell tacos! We stopped by on the way, placed an order of ten regular tacos and ten supreme tacos! Jimmy told the girl at the window that I had just finished my last breast cancer chemotherapy. When our order came out the crew had written Congratulations and decorated both boxes! They all came to the window to give me a thumb up and congratulations! It made me smile even bigger to have such encouragement from total strangers. Also, Jimmy would be able to cook and grocery shop normally! My Surprise Hair could start growing! Never know what comes in, so I might get curly hair like my sister Lynne. I have always had straight hair. That would be a hoot!

We had so much to look forward to!

My Brain is Back!
Chapter 10

Poor Jimmy has had to live with my limited conversation abilities for months. My brain had become the Dead Zone! He had been my walking calendar, helping me to keep up with what day it was or whether I had an appointment getting close. I had trouble remembering birthdays! I have always been the one who knew everyone's birthday! In fact, for years for Christmas I made calendars with all the birthdays for all our family members. When my brain woke up unfortunately for Jimmy I remembered things that I wanted to discuss. Jimmy said, "It's like watching you wake up from a coma." I especially wanted to talk about our long-distance shooting hobby. Our long-distance shooting is for precision and accuracy at distances of one-half to three-fourths of a mile. Eventually we hope to participate in some competitions. I had to inquire, did he trim the cases? How many times were the cases loaded, etcetera? Normally that is my job to keep track of all the loading details and I had to ask! Best part was his answers, he had done it like I always do! That said it All!

This happened about two weeks after my last infusion. My brain woke up with such gusto that I had trouble sleeping! It became like a geyser! The ideas and information spewed! So many ideas of creative projects I wanted to do for my hobbies. The long-distance shooting, I had ideas on how to load for better distance and accuracy. For my wood carving, an explosion of plans, in fact I started one. With my painting I had to sketch concepts and for sewing I had intricate patterns for quilts. The writing of this book involved many late hours at night when I couldn't sleep because of things I wanted to make sure I got down on paper. I kept thinking that this book had to have all the details that I would have wanted to know for going through the Speed Bump of HER2-positive breast cancer. Talking to friends and family, no one had any experience with this type of breast cancer. The only books I could find were text books.

Jimmy had to listen to all the thoughts coming out of mouth! I am known to babble, but it must have been like walking from a quiet room to a blaring concert! Having my brain back may have been a bit trying for Jimmy, as I kept making up for the last five months. And maybe a little extra!

I do not know why my brain woke up with such gusto. As had been the pattern of the previous infusions, the last of the three weeks between infusions had been my better days. Each time it helped with the encouragement to get the next infusion. Knowing it was the last time to have side effects felt very impowering! I had done what others had told me would be the hard part. The feeling of accomplishment inflated my positive attitude! Pollyanna Positive did cartwheels and cheered! She is my own private enthusiastic cheerleader. Maybe that is why my brain came back with such intensity and speed. Whatever the reason it didn't matter. Jimmy and

I enjoyed seeing the light bulb above my head!

The reality was that I had to still deal with the last of the side effects. Love using the word Last! The muffled hearing going away would be fantastic. Not just for me but for everyone who I must tell to talk louder. There are only so many ways to ask someone to repeat something. I have gotten creative about asking. I am sure that no one has noticed that Jimmy talks loudly, so he is easiest to hear!

As expected, I had weakness and had absolutely no stamina. The toes and fingernail tips stayed numb. Additionally, it looked like I may lose both ring fingernails. It would be interesting to see which grows faster, nails or hair? The statistics are that fingernails take six months to grow out and toe nails take up to one and half years. The average for hair regrowth is two to three weeks, a soft fuzz. One to two months, normal thicker hair growth. Two to three months, one inch. Six months of growth should be two to three inches. At twelve months the average is four to five inches of growth.

The side effect that didn't return, the picky, schizophrenic taste buds! They were somewhat numb for a brief time but, I made the list of food to eat that I missed. Examples: DQ Dude, Taco Bell burrito supreme, fried okra and fried chicken. The other list of recipes I planned on making such as: Seafood Newburg, several cold salads, my pot roast, queso and on and on…. I read recipes for entertainment and saved 50 at that point. My sister Lynne found that hilarious!

Cut It Out
Chapter 11

Surgery

I kept doing a post log after my last three weeks with the side effects of chemotherapy. Maybe out of habit, but also to see the progress afterwards. I enjoyed NOT writing some of the side effects!

I felt very good, so we had a mini Opening Weekend. In Texas, it is a tradition on the first weekend of November for the beginning of deer hunting season. Normally it is our big family reunion every year. Even those from out of state try to make it each year. We generally have at least thirty adults and kids! Those who want to hunt, do. They harvest their deer, process it into sausage and share with the rest of the family.

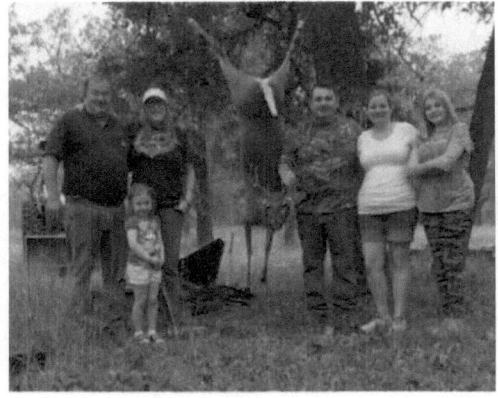

We had Frankie and Jenna and our two granddaughters, Aubrey and Reagan.

They were the only ones we had not seen since before all this started last spring. How wonderful it was to see them after what seemed like a very long time. Aubrey brought me an envelope she had tried to mail to me with get well cards and pictures. It had been returned in the mail, but having her deliver them personally made it even more special. It was particularly unique to have such a small opening weekend but for me it meant more because we did have one. No matter how small Jimmy and I didn't miss the year without having family during a time of tradition. There had been so many things we missed, but not this one. During this weekend Frankie got his first deer and Jimmy got the biggest one he had ever seen. We processed Jimmy's deer into venison steaks. Normally Jimmy and I make venison sausage, steaks and ground venison, but not this year since I could not help. Everyone in the family would still be getting some venison.

Protocol called for surgery, three weeks after the final chemotherapy was completed. From what I have heard from other types of breast cancer protocols, surgery is first, then chemotherapy is second. The steps for surgery are interesting. First, an MRI is done to compare to the one done before chemotherapy. Next, the pin insertion into the center of where the lump originated, while getting an ultrasound for guidance. The pin is a new part of the breast cancer protocol. This is the first and only non-radioactive implant used in wire-free localization. The pin is referred to as a radar breast tumor localization system. It is replacing the wire that has been used for many years. In fact, it had just been approved for placement when the biopsy was taken. This approval happened a couple of days before my insertion. Having that capability, it would save the patient one step before surgery. It would be one of the improvements that is a huge help for the patient. The part I found comical of the whole procedure was that my boob was the center of attention of the technician, radiological doctor, representative for the pin company and myself huddled around the Boob smasher! Another ego boost for my boob as it reminded me of being on Broadway with the center light on it! If anyone had walked in the room they would have thought we were fascinated by something that caught our attention. I remembered how everyone gathers around when we find a weird bug at the ranch that no one has ever seen before! I made jokes about the ego of my right boob. Everyone realized the humor of it from a patient's point of view. The pin has radar for the surgeon to plan the incision and estimate the area for removal. Then, the scheduled pre-op appointment. My surgeon predicted that it would still be a lumpectomy and the removal of several lymph nodes. All that we did in a week! I was exhausted and glad for a break!

November 15th, the Day of Surgery arrived! Of course, before the surgery we had to go in early to have another radiologist give me four shots of radioactive salt solution to light up the road map from the tumor to the lymph nodes.

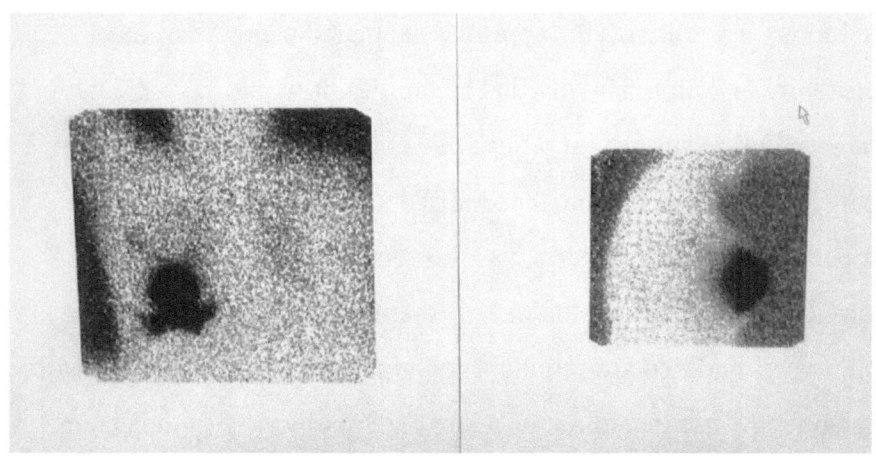

This is a picture of the scan.

This is a Radioisotope test, par for the course, I had to have another set of pictures taken in a specific amount of time to view the road map. After all the pictures and attention, I was sure that my right boob was getting an inflated ego again! My boob probably imagined the paparazzi! Everyone had to get a picture.

Finally, time to get ready for surgery scheduled for noon. No more tests, just an IV placement. We had the meet-and-greet with each of the Surgery Team. I still had not met a single person that isn't full of smiles, positive attitudes and genuine care for the patient and their family. Everyone we meet is intrigued about Alpine. Especially those that don't know there are mountains in Texas! We were again amazed at their curiosity of the side effects I had experienced while on chemotherapy. The remnants of the boils being obvious, which is how the conversation started. These were the best people in their field and yet, as I went through the various stages of my protocol it was surprising how curious everyone is about the other steps of the protocol. That became another reason to write the book for not only the patient and caregivers. My hope is that those in the field will learn of the experience of a patient has during all the steps of this protocol.

Showtime! Took a ride to the operating room! YES! My excitement showed as I kept babbling ninety to nothing. I scooted onto the operating table, which I must say is kind of weird. It was so narrow compared to the bed I road in on that it reminded me of a surf board! I guess that is not odd since I grew up in Corpus Christi. Then I saw the nurse with a shot headed for the IV. I asked, "Is that the night-night juice?" I never heard her answer ...... Time Warp!

In the waiting room Jimmy noticed when my surgeon walked out smiling. He said, "It must have gone good, you are smiling." She said that the tumor had been removed but it had become a calcified sack. Cancer killing juice from chemotherapy had worked very well! Lymph nodes showed no signs of cancer from MRI and visually. She removed one node for pathology verification. Much better news than we could have ever expected. Jimmy understood her smile from ear to ear!

My next vision was of Jimmy. Evidently, I had been trying to wake up telling Jimmy "I missed you." All together now. Awhhhhh. I recovered from the anesthesia quickly and ready to get my clothes on to get going. I know that I asked Jimmy to repeat the surgery results at least three times. Then it sunk in at the wonderful news. To say we felt relieved is an understatement. The step of surgery may have taken a shorter amount of time but had as much importance as the chemotherapy!

The recovery from the surgery was minimal. I experienced soreness as expected, but as for pain, a surprisingly a short amount of time. I only needed the pain medication occasionally for the first two days afterwards. On the third day after surgery, Saturday, the phone rang. To my surprise it was my surgeon calling, she had gotten the pathology report. The results showed no remaining cancer cells! I love that she called us as soon as she got it. Waiting for those types of tests results can loom over your head waiting for a business day. A week later I saw my surgeon for the post operation appointment. She said my progress after surgery looked good. The surgery did not leave a big crater, in fact I would call it a small dimple if you knew the location.

Time for the next appointment with my oncologist and my first Trastuzumab (Herceptin®)-only infusion. Protocol calls for Trastuzumab (Herceptin®) only infusions to start three weeks after surgery. That infusion had side effects of diarrhea for three days. The stomach gave me some trouble, some dizziness and very tired. The fatigue remained a part of each day. I felt that some of the side effects were enhanced because it had been such a short amount of time from chemotherapy. My body probably did a double take at receiving the Trastuzumab (Herceptin®).

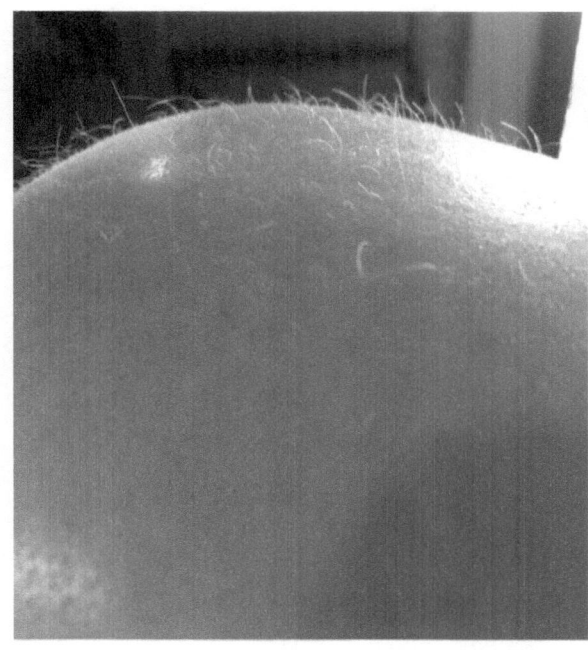

My hair growth had started ever so slightly. No matter how little, I was just happy to see any progress. As you can tell in the picture we had to use a flashlight to see it! Jimmy made sure that I saw the progress!

Both my surgeon and oncologist gave me the all clear to travel. Thank goodness with Thanksgiving being right around the corner! What a fantastic trip home! Aaron sent me food treats from their food truck. He sent fried okra with everything, my favorite! Not only did we get to see our family there but to be home and to feel closer to normal felt refreshing. Nice not having to worry so much about my white count. We could not stay long, but it was worth it seeing all the beauty of fall in Alpine. It is so gorgeous!

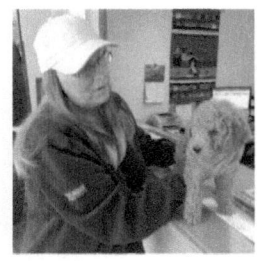

While home I even made it out to see the new puppy my friend Wilma had gotten.

Radiotherapy?
Can I have Classic Rock?
Chapter 12

Beginning of December, time for the temperatures to fall. First, the next step in my protocol, Trastuzumab (Herceptin®)-only infusions every three weeks. This would be until the end of June that is my full-year date since I had my first infusion July sixth. The side effects of just the Trastuzumab (Herceptin®) involved some diarrhea, extremely tired, dizziness, a few stomach issues and a little of the heavy head. These effects in no way had near the intensity of the chemotherapy! I just kept reminding myself that behind the side effects also included the after effects that would be diminishing over the next year or so. One interesting thing happened, one day I threw up for no reason at all. I did not have stomach cramps, nausea, food poisoning and I was not pregnant! Afterwards I felt better. It made no sense, but I didn't care.

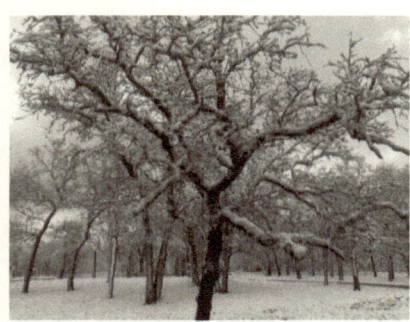

It snowed at the ranch the day after my infusion! How astonishing since we do not get snow there but once every ten years!

The first week after the infusion proved a bit difficult, but at least I had a beautiful view out my window!

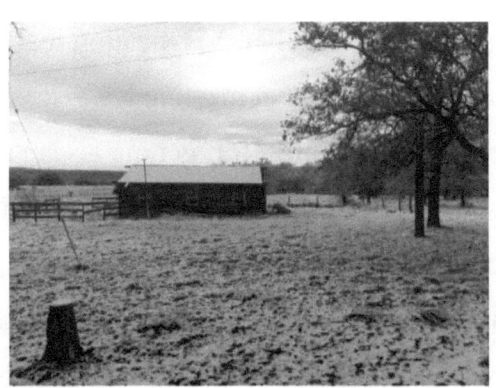

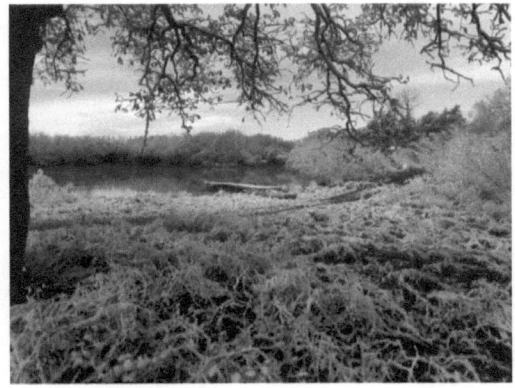

Next, the appointment with my Radiation Oncologist. Radiotherapy is another term used for radiation therapy. The first thought for me-music. Get it Radiotherapy? Some of the terms used either make my eyes roll in the back of my head or giggle to myself. My radiation oncologist looked at the results from the surgery and pathology, after which he explained the path for me. The results showed that with the chemotherapy the cancer had a (PCR) Pathological Complete Response! Which in Kaye talk means, "The Chemotherapy completely kicked my cancers buttocks into oblivion!" The incredible part is how I knew it was working after the second chemotherapy treatment. Hearing that gave Jimmy and I a huge feeling of relief. Verification that Boob Cancer had been knocked out! In that meeting we discussed the radiation treatments that I would qualify for, getting a scan to map out the target area while also getting markers placed. Then we would be starting. If the scan showed that I qualified for the pin point radiation it would mean sixteen treatments instead of twenty-eight regular radiation treatments. There would be four special-boost radiation treatments also. That added up to twenty sessions instead of twenty-eight. I could not have been more thrilled about that! Less time in the medical tanning booth!

The new machine he had told us about on our previous appointment had still been scheduled to be online January first. If I qualified, which he felt very confident of, we could not start till January. The Christmas holidays were coming soon also, so we decided to wait.

The scan was scheduled to check my qualifying and to place the markers. The objective of the scan is also placing the dots for alignment during radiation. These dots are like getting three tiny tattoos. They are made permanent so that when receiving the radiation, it is aligned to correctly target the area for the radiation.

All we had left to do, check with my oncologist to see if we could push the next Trastuzumab (Herceptin®) infusion one week to be able to spend the holidays at home. He had no problem with postponing till the beginning of January. Check, check we had the all clear after the scan to go home for the holidays!

I had decorated a Christmas tree, set out some of my

nutcrackers and added other touches for Christmas to have the holidays at the ranch. We did not know if we would be able to go home however, it would be another nice break to be back for winter in Alpine. No need for an excuse for a fire in the fireplace type of weather. We were going to be able to spend a wonderful Christmas Eve with the kids and grandkids.

My hair had been growing for two months now. It may not seem like much to anyone else but to me, a strong beginning of my new hair with an oddity.

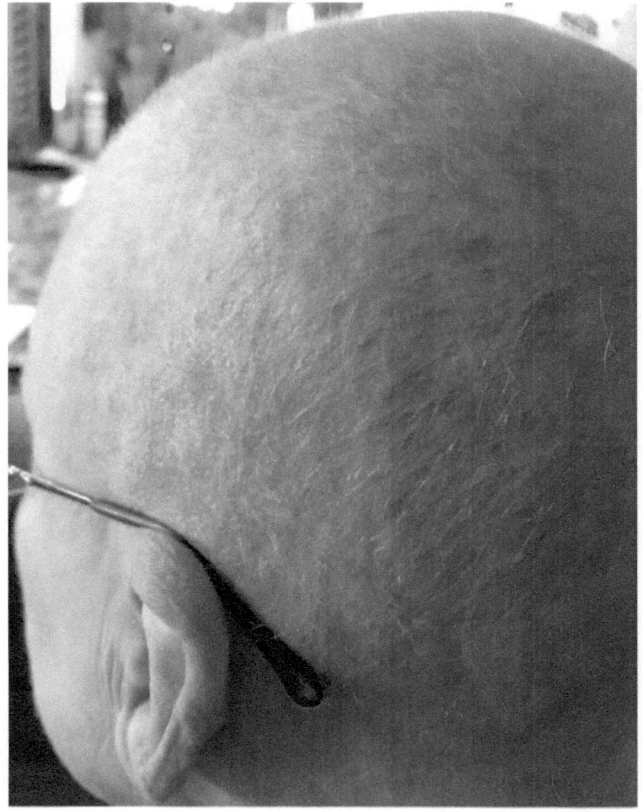

The oddity was it grew faster on the left side of my head. Uhmmm, I couldn't figure out why. This happened to be one of the things as my hair grew that continued.

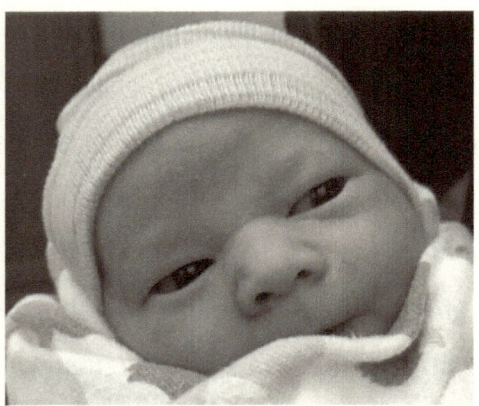

We also had a blessing arrive before Christmas, the birth of our great grandson. Yes, life goes on while you are fighting cancer, thank goodness. Knowing this gave me even more reason to finish and get back to our life and family!

We had a wonderful time while at home. Our stay ended up being for only ten days but better than not being able to take a break. Now, time to get back to my job of completing the protocol!

Will I Glow or Tan?
Chapter 13

Sixteen Pin Point Radiation Treatments

The beginning of January, the start of a new year. Time to get started on the radiation treatments. Just like chemotherapy, there is a learning curve of the side effects. It would be sixteen daily treatments followed by four daily booster treatments. Since I had a Complete Response from the chemotherapy, I qualified for the new machine that is pin point radiation. In other words, only my Boob will glow in the dark! Seriously, not having it radiate the other parts of my upper body, I could not have been more appreciative.

On Wednesday, January third began my radiation treatments, they were very short. I spent more time to undress and dress! The technicians Kim and Kimberly were fabulous! They talked me through every step no matter how minor. I immediately looked forward to seeing them every day I went in. When you start radiation, it is every week-day. We would chat before getting my treatment and after, for a minute or two. During my third treatment while chatting, I told them that I had HER2-positive Boob Cancer. Just like other medical personnel they had a curiosity about the side effects of my chemotherapy treatment. Then I learned that one of them had a relative who found out she had another kind of Boob

Cancer. I told her I started writing a book to tell my story and experiences. Also told her about the Chemo Care Baskets that I suggested before starting. I offered to print a copy of it for her relative. She could help her relative by getting some of the basics that might be needed before she began. This experience gave me additional reasons to keep writing.

While doing radiation therapy they recommend putting lotion or cream on your breast. This is SO Important! They will tell you which brands they suggest. They gave me a sample of Calendula cream. I put the cream on at least three times a day. It turned out to be essential during my radiation treatments, in fact I ended up ordering two more tubes! Do not be hesitant about using it.

I had a weekend break after my first three treatments. The side effects in the beginning were like a sunburn. I am very lucky to have skin that doesn't react to the sun most of the time I will get a little pink but by bedtime I am tan. Anyone like my sister Lynne would have had a much harder time because of sensitivity. She is fairer skinned and sensitive to sun burns and dryness. Besides feeling like being out in the sun, itching also occurred. I am heavy breasted which seemed to create more irritation under my boob even though my lump had been located on the top of my boob. Again, the lotion helped with everything! The drive to go every day for the treatments took about forty-five minutes to go to Kyle. When we went in for infusions in Round Rock it generally took one and one-half hours if the traffic cooperated!

On the day of my second radiation treatment I also had my

---

next Trastuzumab (Herceptin®) infusion. We knew that it had been a breakthrough drug for HER2-positive. The statistics are amazing! Jimmy had been reading about how Trastuzumab (Herceptin®) is now on the World Health Organizations Model List of Essential Medicines. This list contains the medications considered to be the most effective and safe to meet the most important needs in a health system. Trastuzumab (Herceptin®) was added along with fifteen other cancer medicines. The protocol for HER2-positive is a full year of infusions of Trastuzumab (Herceptin®). This meant that I would have infusions for the next six months to my one-year mark. These Trastuzumab (Herceptin®) infusions are an essential part of doing the most you can to keep your body's defenses up against HER2-positive. Besides any medical reasoning, I know that it will prevent any cells from multiplying, preventing any cancer growth. In Kaye talk, it means, "If there is one stupid or stubborn cell hanging around this will knock it flat!" Or you could call it CYA protocol!

The side effects were not near the impact as those of the chemotherapy! The fatigue from the chemotherapy is accentuated by the Trastuzumab (Herceptin®). There is the irritated nasal passages and a cough. This time I did have one day of diarrhea. Jimmy and I were both relieved that it materialized for just one day! Dizziness still occurred occasionally.

We had tremendous love and support from family and friends that had an influence that can only be described as immeasurable! I had not shed a tear since we found out that I had Boob Cancer, because I knew it would not win against me! I did shed many smiles and felt the warmth in my heart from all the support.

The following week would be the next five radiation treatments. By the end of that week I appreciated being half way through the sixteen pin point treatments. Getting through the first eight treatments is something to feel good about. It was the point I began to see some of the side effects. Now, going every day can be a bit tiring. It had only been about ten weeks since finishing the chemotherapy. Naps being a part of each day, in fact many times I would fall asleep on the ride home from the treatments.

At this point it had been about two and one-half months since my last chemotherapy infusion. I began to be able to say, "I am feeling good" and mean it when I felt good!

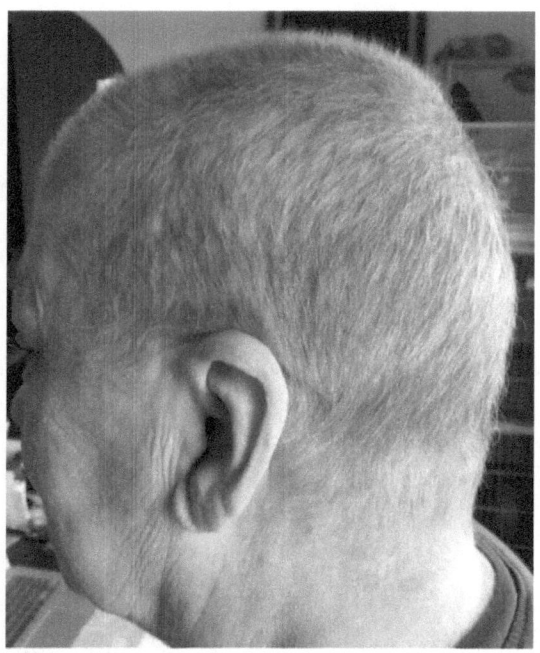

My hair maintained its growth fast and furiously. At 3 months it had black, grey and blonde or light brown. I guess you could call it Calico hair!

The eyebrows were back in black, about ¼ inch long and Very Full Eyelashes are surprisingly coming in fuller than before! Astonishingly the body hair had not even started. I had the quiet wish that my leg hair would forget how to grow and not come back! My legs are long and I could save on buying razors. That would be a great gift. I did notice at this point since starting infusions seven months ago that my adult acne had ceased to exist. Adult acne had been a part of my whole adult life but not at all during my teenage years. It never got severe, just annoying. Especially when an event was approaching, my face would breakout with a pimple that felt as obvious as a clown's nose. I had been so focused on the cancer treatment that the disappearance of acne went quietly away like a sailboat in the night. When I realized this, I ran down the hallway to the kitchen announcing loudly to Jimmy, "My Acne is Gone! My Acne is Gone!" He was shocked that neither one of us had observed the change. Strike a point for Pollyanna Positive! I kept my fingers crossed and hoped that it did not come back with time.

After my second weekend break, time for my ninth treatment. At the beginning of the first eight treatments, simple as I said, like getting some sun then back to normal the next morning. By the ninth treatment I started getting some very itchy areas and additional redness that stayed day-to-day. On the day of my tenth treatment I got an unexpected break. A snow and ice storm came to central Texas again! This made the third snow in central Texas in one winter. It is so abnormal for this area! The poor residents of the area have no experience for driving in these types of conditions. It works better to just tell everyone to stay home! We got the call from the radiation office that they had closed due to weather. I felt like a kid with school being cancelled! Put on a movie and make some popcorn!

We resumed my tenth treatment on the following day, Tuesday. With starting the eleventh treatment on Thursday, large blisters started developing under my breast. After the twelfth treatment on Friday we were getting very concerned about the skin under my boob. The blisters started breaking open to raw skin. They became red, irritated and very raw! Some bumps broke out above my boob that itched like crazy! I tried to go to the grocery store with Jimmy but realized that I couldn't do it before we got to the door. The dizziness and exhaustion gave me fits. It turned out to be obvious the radiation added to the fatigue. I still had some issues with being light headed from Herceptin® infusions too.

To keep the area dry under my breast we tried keeping it lifted to keep dry. That was a challenge! The mechanisms we tried were done by trial and error. Imagine trying to hold up one boob and not letting anything touch underneath! First idea, the bathing suit top with string ties, that lasted a couple of hours. Next, the lop-sided modifications to a bra. That lasted one day till the modifications broke. Jimmy created the final and lasting solution. He took one of his old rifle slings and modified it to hold the breast high and steady in place! I guess you could have called me a boob slinger! It worked great! It was Not fashionable, but because of the relief I did not give a flip about how I looked! My boob stayed up and let the air get to it!

Realize that I had to also wear a long-sleeve open button-up shirt to keep the air available and button up in case someone dropped by and to keep me from getting cold.

We felt relieved to have the weekend break to try to help get the issues under some sort of control. I also started alternating Caladryl, triple antibiotic and baby powder to keep it dry and help heal too. By the thirteenth treatment on Monday it looked better below my boob, but the bumps above increased in number as did the itching. Then began the break out of pus pockets that popped up all over my breast. They generally were small and busted when I slept.

I had an appointment on Tuesday with my radiology oncologist at the fourteenth treatment. He said that he would not delay my treatment and would give me medication if needed for the issues I experienced under my breast. It calmed me that I would be able to continue.

After the fifteenth and sixteenth regular pin point treatments my breast stayed red. On Thursday, was the sixteenth treatment. One of the other things I started using at this point was ice cubes. I would run the ice cube on my bumps on the top of my boob to help with the itch and irritation, drying afterwards. I did not let the water get under my boob and even didn't use the lotion under my boob. Moisture below hindered healing underneath.

One of the things I noticed at this time, the deterioration of my finger nails looked like they seemed to be getting better. Keeping them short helped. Unfortunately, while concentrating on the radiation treatments I neglected to keep them trimmed.

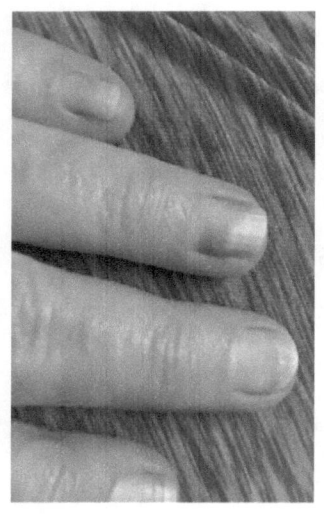
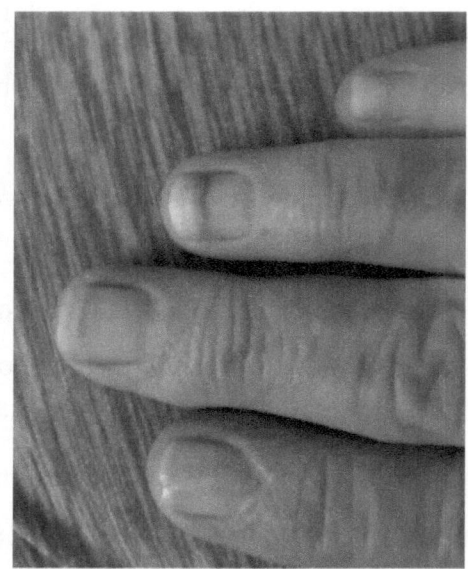

Here are pictures of them and
a break that could have been very painful.

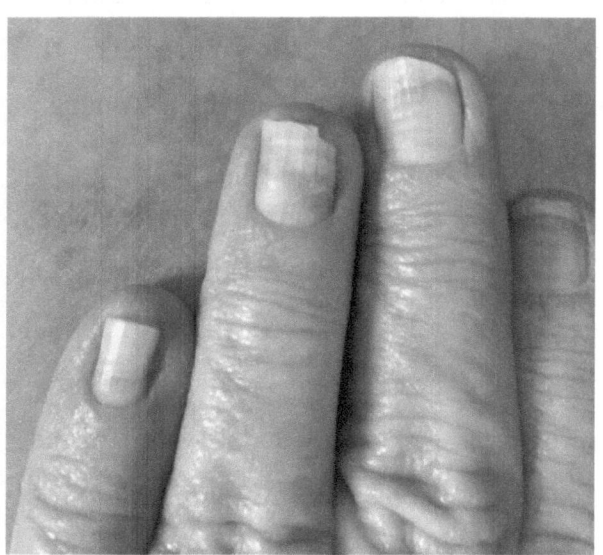

I also had my scheduled Trastuzumab (Herceptin®) infusion
on the same day of my sixteenth treatment of radiation. I spoke to
my oncologist about the dizziness. If I got up fast, I had to sit back
down. Dizziness would happen immediately. It was happening

frequently. Also happened when I would try to walk into the grocery store or walk into the house from the car. He gave me a prescription for Meclizine. It helped, especially the first week after the infusion. The heavy head hung around for two weeks after the infusion and fatigue. Only had diarrhea for one day, thank goodness! The rest of the infusions we considered as follow up. Jimmy said, "You had been a good cooperative patient." It was good to hear that because I had tried throughout everything to do my best at each step of the protocol. Jimmy had also told me every night, "You are my girl" and I would tell him, "You are my prince." It kept my spirit high while losing my hair, skin color, energy and the general feeling of looking in the mirror and not seeing me. My Prince had been an Outstanding Caregiver! He had been there for all the good, bad and the ugly part of battling Boob Cancer. With Jimmy as my caregiver, I didn't need a caretaker!

Becoming Well Done!
Chapter 14

Four Full Radiation Treatments

On Friday, began the start of the last four booster treatments and I became concerned they would postpone the last treatments. These four treatments were full on radiation because my insurance didn't approve the other type of booster. Compared to the pin point treatments there is quite a difference.

After the first of the full-on radiation treatments my boob turned Very Red! We had a weekend break that followed this treatment which ended up being great timing. The full-on radiation created the blisters, itching, discomfort and redness tenfold. I appreciated having only four of those treatments. I never felt the need to ask for a break as the timing of the weekends had been perfect. If you feel you have the need to have a break, ask the doctor. The radiation treatments are more flexible. I could have asked for a break if I felt I needed it. Through the weekend I had trouble sleeping because my boob being sore, and the bumps hurt. Keeping dry underneath at night proved to be a dilemma because of sweating while I slept. I would try to position the covers to keep them off my boob. At one point I folded a paper towel in half and placed it under my boob when I went to bed and changed it during the night when I would wake up. Doing that seemed to help with sweating and the fluid oozing from the raw open blisters. Forget rolling over! That was very hard and PAINFUL! My boob would have screeched if I tried rolling over!

On Monday, time for the second full on treatment. The spot where my lump had been, became deep red. Surprisingly a shower felt very good after this treatment! The water had to run from behind me flowing over my boob. NOT straight on because it felt like hail hitting my boob! The water couldn't be too hot or too cold. It had to be Goldilocks style, just right.

On Tuesday, the third full on treatment. The spot where my lump had been, became brown red. I had found a camisole soft enough to wear under shirts. It became like my security blanket camisole! I slept in it, washed it during coffee in the morning to be able to wear it each day to my treatments! My whole boob being so very tender, I had to wear my security camisole with very light and soft shirts that could in No Way be tight when I went into public. The rest of my boob was deep red now.

January 31st had come! The day the Radiation Is Done! So is my Boob! As in Well Done! On the fourth and final full-on radiation treatment my boob almost said, "I give!" Poor baby looked fully cooked.

As Jimmy and I were getting ready for the appointment for the final radiation treatment, we both thought of what we had done handling this Speed Bump. When I came out from getting dressed

Jimmy gave me the thumbs up. He had calculated the time since the Doctor appointment of setting up more images because the lump looked like it may be serious.

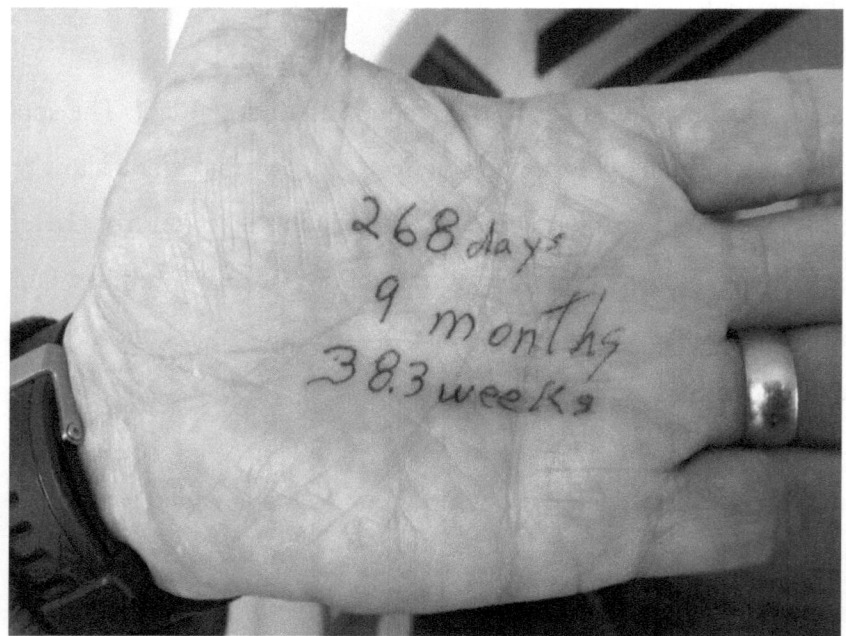

It had been 268 days, 9 months, or 38.3 weeks. Jimmy wrote this in his palm to show when he gave me the thumbs up!

I laughed as again Jimmy encouraged me in another unexpected way! It also helped us realize how long we have worked together to drive over the cancer Speed Bump.

As I have said before, the people of Austin Cancer Center are Wonderful! We were so excited on the way to radiation of the final treatment. I would be done! The excitement of the people at Austin Cancer Center was so much more than I would have ever expected.

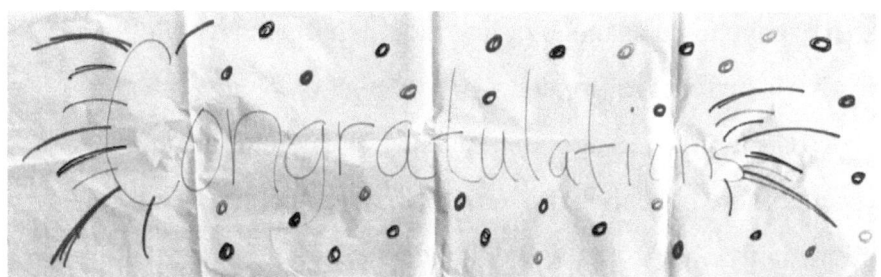

Everyone gave me a thumbs up while congratulating me on my last treatment when we arrived. Kim and Kimberly, my radiation nurses, had put a sign of Congratulations for me on the table I lay on.

Such a Surprise! After I finished we hugged, and they gave me a certificate of finishing signed by all the girls. The support, caring and personal feeling they give to patients is beyond words!

Afterward we went home for the break we had before my next infusion. During that time in Alpine, I still had to sit around letting the air get to the raw skin from the blisters. Sitting around comfortably made it easier than wearing something. One thing we added to my regiment, putting on Neosporin® Pain and Relief Cream. The wonder drug for my Well-Done Boob! Also, my boob was surprisingly swollen! I don't think I could have fit it into my bra. Forget wearing a bra anyway. My boob would have let me know that wasn't happening!

One point I would like to mention is by the time I finished all my steps of beating cancer there were some new studies being done. These involved the radiation part of HER2-positive. There are trials in progress about how much radiation or not needing the radiation. This may be part of a (PCR) Pathological Complete Response. My hope that in the future they may find that not all HER2-positive patients have to do as much or any radiation treatments. Pollyanna Positive is betting it changes!

During the radiation treatments it did add to the fatigue. As expected, I did have the leftovers from chemotherapy. I had been told from my doctors that it would be a year after chemotherapy before I felt back to my normal self before chemotherapy. The peripheral neuropathy of numbness in my feet became part of every day. The other things I experienced included muscle weakness, lack of energy and naps. Jimmy was my go-to guy for opening jars or even emptying ice trays. The funny part, these jars had already been open! The one muscle that kept working overtime, my brain. Jimmy tried to keep up with my babbling and jumping subjects within seconds of a pause in our conversations. He also had to get use to me "correcting" him! We were able to have abundant conversations about our long-distance shooting hobby, cooking with our Sous Vide and even the news! It had been awhile since I could keep up with everything going on in the world! Many of our talks consisted of how we felt it seemed like experiencing a soft landing after chemotherapy and a pathological complete response. Having the last of the Trastuzumab (Herceptin®) infusions would be no problem to handle and do. These are part of the protocol! They are the bow on top of the gift of being cured. As Jimmy said, "You can't be un-cured!" Quote of the day, maybe of the year.

Staying on the Infusion Road
Chapter 15

After finishing my radiation treatments, we transitioned part time at home, not full time at the ranch.

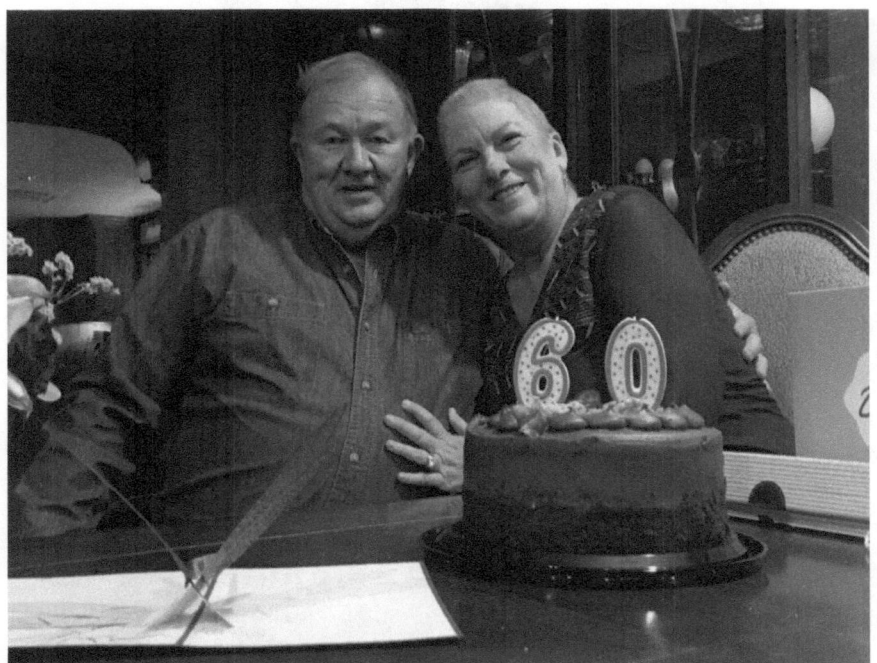

Right before we headed back to the ranch I had my sixtieth birthday. Jimmy and I spent a wonderful evening celebrating my 60th Birthday and Cancer Free!

The progress of my hair at four months of growth was coming along very well. I could not help but be pleased as it seemed to be coming in as thick as I had before.

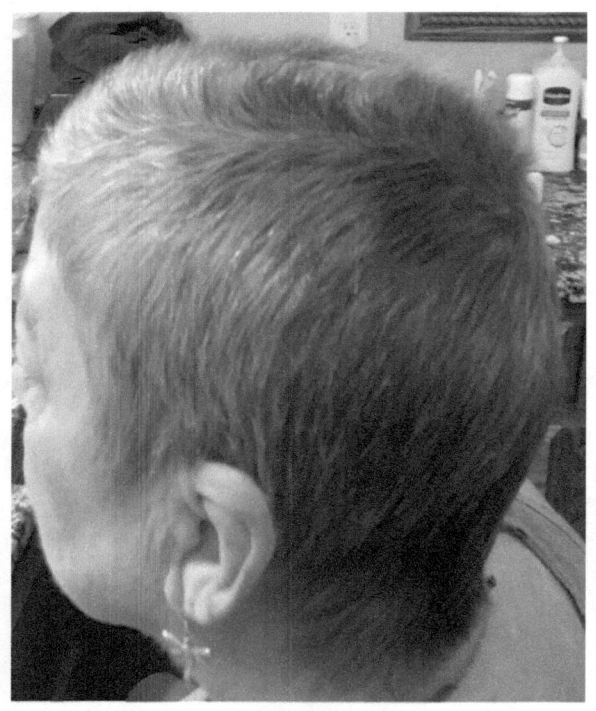

The colors looked light black, dark brown and grey.

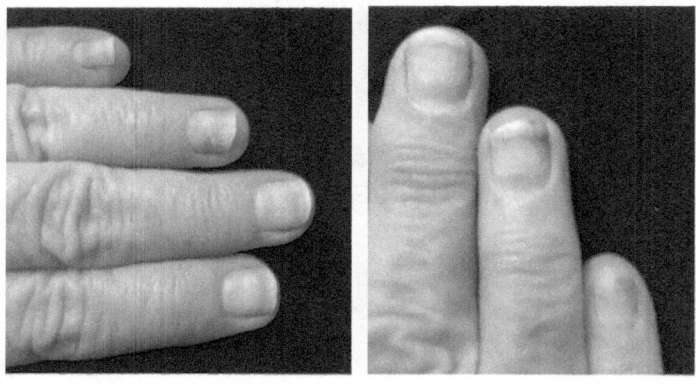

Also, my finger nails were looking much better.

At the two weeks mark after radiation, we had a follow-up with my radiology oncologist. My doctor liked seeing the progress made since the last treatment. Unfortunately, the side effects of the radiation treatments turned out to be much more than I had expected as time went on. The tenderness became so sensitive that wearing only very soft shirts remained the only option when I wasn't sitting around topless with only an open button up shirt. Sleeping kept being difficult. Turning over or shifting in my sleep at night kept being very painful. The blisters continued to come to the surface and break creating more tender spots. I think my boob felt embarrassed to sit around topless because it looked terrible and would have made people cringe. If I had to sit around topless I am sure that my boob would prefer to look beautiful like usual! My boob skin was tight, swollen, red, blistered, pus pockets and raw for about two weeks after the last treatment. Thank goodness I had my security camisole!

It was now the beginning of March. Time for the next scheduled Trastuzumab (Herceptin®) infusion. I have some advice about being at this point of the protocol. I know that you become tired of appointments, being poked and prodded but keep going! Don't Stop before this Race is Over! Make sure to take control of your schedule. If you must get something else done or test, do the logistics to have any other things the same week of your infusion. It is time to try to get back part of a normal life.

Jimmy and I began starting the count down to the last of the infusions. After this infusion I would have only five more to go! Woohoo! It is such a brief time at the infusion, about thirty minutes after starting the bag. With this Trastuzumab (Herceptin®) infusion the side effect of fatigue did not diminish. I had to keep reminding myself that these were partially left over from the chemotherapy.

The naps seemed to be shorter but almost a daily occurrence. On the fourth day afterward, I threw up for no reason at all and felt better afterwards again. The dizziness and heavy head persisted off and on for about two weeks. The medication (Meclizine) the doctor prescribed, and ibuprofen helped with both the dizziness and heavy head. The dizziness developed severely enough that Jimmy took precautions to stay close to me in case I went down. Fortunately, I could catch the dizzy spell each time by sitting back down. Then another side effect happened that surprised me! I started waking up every morning blowing my nose. Now that doesn't sound surprising to most, but, I started having boogers galore! Then I started having blood coming with my nose blowing in the morning. I do not have allergies like many people, so this blew me away! Sorry for that pun, I know it was a groaner. The other thing I noticed, my throat seemed a little irritated, not sore, just sensitive. At this point I assumed that these had to be side effects of the nasal passages, throat and sinuses. Of course, from previous experience of the chemotherapy, I know that this may or may not show up after the next infusion. Life in the year of the cancer Speed Bump has been full of surprises!

Radiation Surprises!
Chapter 16

Late March, time for the next infusion. I started coming to grips with the length of time it would take me to get back to my young self. With the continuation of the Trastuzumab (Herceptin®) infusions and the side effects, I knew I would not start getting over all the side effects until July. That is the beginning of the year recovery according to the doctors. Of course, I planned on doing it in record time!

Then came the break out of what I call "Surprise Blisters" from the radiation. It had been about two months from the end of the radiation. They had been hiding under the skin waiting to catch me off guard. It would look like a big red spot on my boob at first. Then they would get Very Sore. As they got larger and extremely tender I became concerned. While dressing one morning one of them busted. I didn't realize they were pustules so to my surprise filled with pus. I had to start the hydrogen peroxide, triple antibiotic ointment and band aid routine. They looked too much like the boils, so I became very alarmed. One of the things that seemed odd and kind of unsettling, these Surprise Blister came from under an area where the swelling looked odd. The areas that I had stretch marks were very extended with the swelling. That is where the Surprise Blisters came out. My thoughts immediately, in those areas the skin was thinner. Who knows!

The appointment for the follow-up with my surgeon, is where she relieved my concerns. She said that my progress looked good and told me not to be alarmed by the blister breakout. We discussed having corrective surgery to fix the issues of balance and change of the right breast. When I looked at my breast I would think of a teeter totter with my left breast on the ground and my right breast up in the air! My surgeon gave me the name of a plastic surgeon to meet with concerning that surgery. It could not be done until five months after radiation, which would be July. I couldn't imagine doing it before fall as it needs time for the left overs from radiation to heal, soften and return to somewhat normal. She also said that I would be scheduled for a digital 3-D mammogram in May. From what she said this mammogram will count as my yearly for both breasts but, my right breast will get one in six months. These are becoming more popular and find lumps sooner.

At my appointment with my oncologist I had become accustomed to hearing my blood counts. This time I realized that I still enjoyed hearing the results. Maybe out of habit with it being critical during chemotherapy. While meeting with my oncologist we discussed when the port would be removed. I wanted to know mostly out of curiosity. The port is no problem, in fact, I am not anxious to have it removed. He said that it would probably be one year after my last infusion. I would have to get my port flushed every four to six weeks during that year, preferably every four weeks.

Our biggest issues were my fatigue and dizziness. Maybe some brain fog, but Jimmy is thankful when it subsides and I start babbling profusely! The changes created nick names. The first week after the Trastuzumab (Herceptin®) I became Dodo head. The second week I became Groot. At that point Jimmy could ask me to bring a wrench and I would have brought him a banana. Everyone thought it was hilarious. I did too because I could never tell what my reaction might be. Conversations turned into laughter most of the time!

The nasal, drainage and throat issues continued with the dry nasal passages, boogers and bloody nose. It did seem to subside after two weeks. Fatigue also seemed to be less but still had some consistency of needing naps occasionally.

During the whole process of getting over the Speed Bump of Boob Cancer we talked about "Climbing out the Window." I had my wildlife garden to see outside my window where I sat. It had been a joy with all the things Jimmy kept adding out there. It also instigated my thinking of a window to see what I will be doing after I finished. I had not mentioned these thoughts to Jimmy. Then one day Jimmy told me how he thought of me looking out a window to my future and climbing out of it! I was amazed that we had the same visions of our future. Of course, it happens quite often as we have been married 37 years. To help me along with "Climbing out the Window," Jimmy bought me a travel trailer to start getting out again! Jimmy and I have always enjoyed RVing, it is our favorite way to travel. He had seen my urge to return to normal and the stumbling blocks I must deal with. It can be disappointing to not be able to do what is normal for yourself. The Prince that he is, Jimmy saw the need to help me keep that from happening! I may not be able to Climb out the Window yet. But I sure as hell can Climb into the RV!!

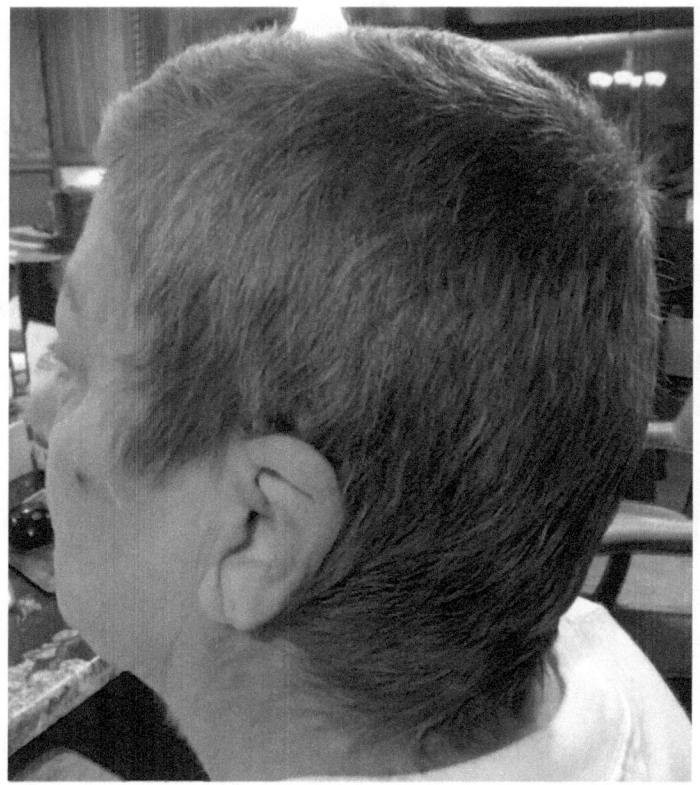

The hair growth kept me smiling from ear to ear! It changed almost daily. Some days at this point it curled, some days it is straight and flat as a board.

I kept looking in the mirror one day wondering why one section of hair stood up and wouldn't lay down. Jimmy walked in asking "What are you looking at?" I pointed to the spot on my head. I said, "Isn't that weird?" Jimmy started laughing telling me that I had a cow-lick! I don't know if it is new or not since I always had long hair, so I never saw it. To try to keep in under control, I began trying to use a product which I have no experience with!

The Countdown
Chapter 17

It was the middle of April, time for the next infusion. The Trastuzumab (Herceptin®) treatments aren't hard, maybe just irritating. To feel so close and yet it seems so far from being finished. Knowing that we are making progress on finishing the protocol is the biggest encouragement. I really enjoyed the week before the infusion, it was the time that I could see what the beginning of my world would be after all the Trastuzumab (Herceptin®) treatments. During that week I did do some of the normal things that I was looking forward to getting back to. It has been enjoyable to go do some long-distance shooting, some wood carving and planning some new quilts! It was Spring, and the wild flowers seemed to be more numerous than normal. I love all the colors and varieties! This is normally when I would have worked in the back yard and planted a garden. We have a wonderful friend, Glen, who had been working on my back yard in Alpine to bring it back to life. He brought everything back to its spring beauty! The roses and wine cups are my favorites and first to begin the explosion of color.

At this point I had the nasal irritation of lots of boogers, some bloody nose and lots of phlegm. The sensitivity to stuffy air and air filled with pollen, sand or hot is stronger. This sensitivity results in a coughing fit and throwing up. Most of the time it happens at the most inopportune time, so I have had to miss several events that I wanted to be at. There were two relatives that passed away at this time. I couldn't attend their funerals that I desperately wanted to go to. The diarrhea and throwing up for no reason happened occasionally for one day. The reliable daily fatigue. As I have been told and mentioned, it will be part of the year recovery although it still had days right then that seemed more intense right after the Trastuzumab (Herceptin®) infusions. My naps didn't last hours long like they were during chemotherapy. I generally laid down and slept for about an hour. When I was raising my children, I always yawned during the family videos. I learned to do a form of power naps before they became popular. It became a joke that mommy would ask the kids to let me rest my eyes for twenty minutes and yet I would correct them while resting my eyes! Moms have amazing abilities that constantly surprise children!

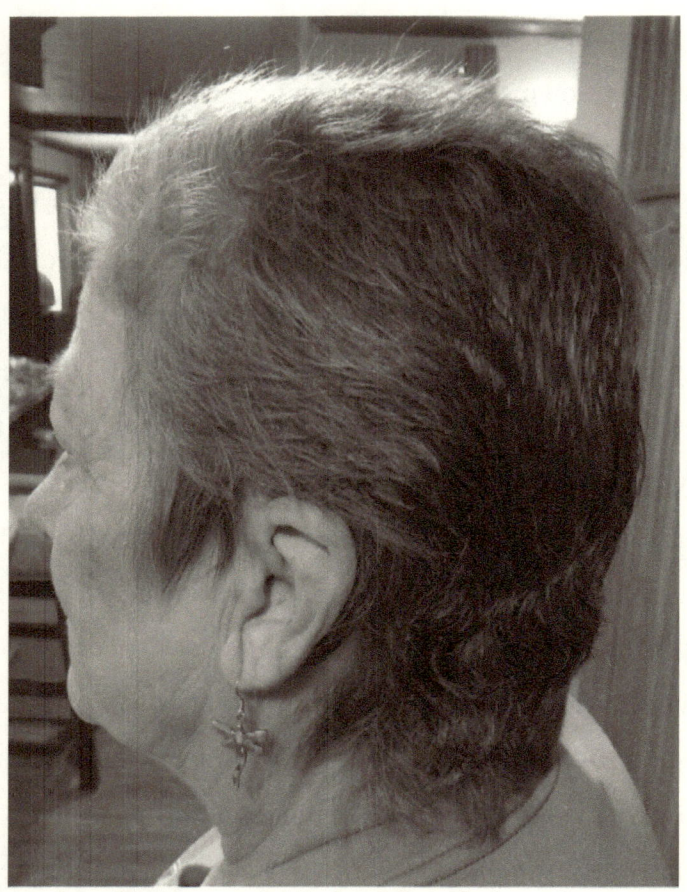

Six months of hair growth! It dumbfounded me the amount of change every month! The feeling of my hair on the back of my neck was heaven. It is the only way to have that constant reminder it is longer! I could not help getting excited!

With this Trastuzumab (Herceptin®) infusion it left three more to go! The biggest part of finishing that I was going to miss was seeing all the friends I had made at Austin Cancer Center. Of course, we had encouraged everyone to come out to Alpine to see the magnificence of West Texas! After we finished getting the infusion, time to have the appointment with the plastic surgeon. As I have breast implants I am very familiar with breast augmentation.

The meeting mostly focused on what could be done when enough time had passed after the radiation. As I mentioned earlier, it could not be done before July. The doctor would be able to be more specific about the surgery according to how my breast had changed by that time. Having corrective surgery is not limited to when it is possible. There is no reason to do it immediately. I decided to wait and see how my breast changed. Remember part of this decision is you knowing your body and how you feel about your body. I felt that by the following fall or next year I would know when or if time had come to consider having the corrective surgery. Partially, the reason for my decision was to let my breast have enough time to see what the full effect between the two would be.

Mammogram Time Again
Chapter 18

I had been scheduled for my yearly mammogram. A digital mammogram, many more pictures than the normal mammogram. Turn this way, turn that way, now the other one. Then another technician had to come in and take other specific pictures. What is funny about going through all these steps of killing Boob Cancer is feeling like you are constantly going to Mardi Gras! Lift your blouse, take off your blouse and bra (or security camisole), put on this paper sack cover or put on a cover that reminded me of going to my hairdresser except I had no hair. Being timid about showing my boob went away very quickly in the beginning of this journey. Everyone I had an appointment with was going to have to look, touch or take a picture my boob. They should give out beads!

Onward on the infusion train. The start of May, time for the next infusion the day after the mammogram. We arrived at the doctor's office ready to begin the normal routine. Our doctor had changed offices, so we weren't at the office I had done all my previous infusions. An issue that we had not been aware of came to the attention of the medical team. I needed to get an echocardiogram before I got my next infusion. Hence the infusion did not happen, and an appointment was made for the echocardiogram. I felt a little disappointed, which may sound surprising but then I realized my clear head would be staying around longer. It ended up showing me more of what to expect to experience after I finished all the rest of the infusions.

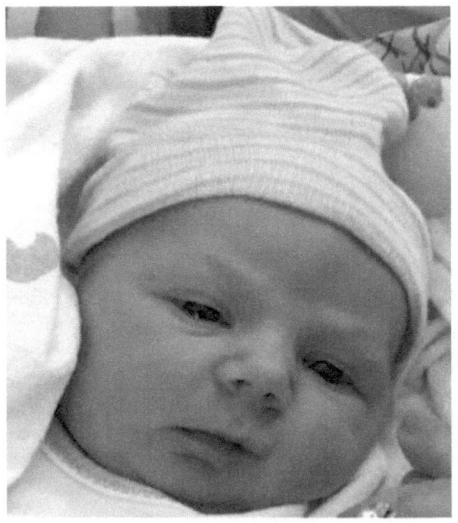

During this time, we had another blessing to our family. The birth of another Granddaughter. Another event that I wish we could have dropped everything to go see her. We did get to meet her at four weeks old. So precious.

The echocardiogram had been scheduled to be done at a hospital. I find it humorous that everywhere else we had scheduled appointments we were given times that easily worked with the drive into Austin. Whenever we have to go to a hospital for a test they can only schedule you first thing in the morning! I am Not a morning person! While raising the kids, I always got up at five thirty every morning getting everyone dressed, brush or braid their hair and having breakfast ready. I did tell everyone that I would sleep when they grew up. I have followed thru and have added two cups of coffee. I didn't discover the magic of coffee until my late thirties. Discovering this nectar of the gods has been part of every day or rather mornings since then.

At seven months of growth most people were amazed at how much my hair had grown. Still trying different ways to style it. Also needing to use a hearing aid occasionally.

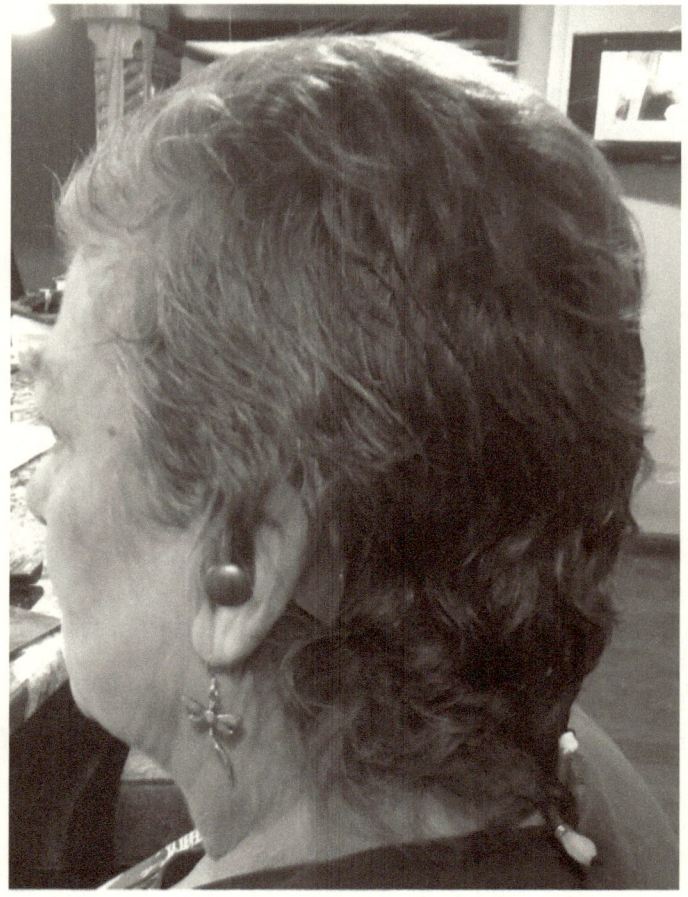

Therefore, ever morning the experiment of styling I found it to be a challenge as my experience is with long hair! It looked so good that I didn't feel like a Chia Pet anymore!

Feeling like a Kid at Christmas
Chapter 19

Here we go, the next to the last infusion! It filled me with
excitement to think about my bounce back after the last infusion. In
some ways like being a kid again on Christmas Eve. Knowing that it
was going to be Christmas soon! Looking forward to opening The
Window, breathing the fresh air and creating the experiences we
would have. Climbing out that window to normal life and wonderful
times with Jimmy.

As I have said throughout this book, I consider my port one
of the best things done before chemotherapy. These thoughts at this
next to last infusion had me wondering how many times it saved me
from getting an IV and kept my veins healthy. It had continued to
make it easier with the blood draws for the blood test and the
Trastuzumab (Herceptin®) infusions. I started to calculate how
many times I saved getting an IV. Then I told myself, "Don't count,
just be thankful missy!" I am in no rush to have it removed. It has
almost become my Speed Bump badge. One other thought I kept
having was how unlike the hormonal breast cancers, I would not
have to take hormone blockers for years. Another addition to the be
thankful list!

The Blood tests came back good, so off to the infusion room

after a visit with my oncologist. When we walked in, a patient had a reaction to the medication. If that happens, everyone is on deck to help. Should this happen while you are in the infusion room remember to have patience, if it happened to you they would be giving you the attention needed. They gave him a shot and within a few minutes he felt normal. Of all my times in an infusion room we only saw this happen three times. Of those three times only one patient had to be sent to the emergency room.

I had also become spoiled to the thirty-minute infusions. It had become such a quick time that I could not even to take a nap. Partially because I knew it would be done before I had time to check email and social media on my tablet. While sitting there I kept thinking of how I had seen all the changes in my body from the end of chemotherapy every day. I enjoyed eating and flavors again which was heaven for me even before breast cancer. Now to know that the next time I sat in this chair for thirty minutes would be my last and it was thrilling to think about.

Jimmy had also introduced me to a Mocha Frappuccino that we could get in Luling, a small town near the ranch. When we had a special occasion or celebration for a mile marker in killing cancer, he would take a detour back from Austin to get me one! Well, since it had been my next to last infusion and the infusion time went so quickly, I asked for the Mocha Frappuccino detour! Imagine my surprise when he walked out with Two of them! Perfect way to end infusion day!

Last but not Least
Chapter 20

Final Trastuzumab (Herceptin®) Infusion

As I sat there at the ranch, looking out my window to the beautiful Wildlife Garden that Jimmy created for me, I couldn't help but think about this last year. It was softly overcast with the drops of the previous rain dripping off the trees. The birds and squirrels were coming in and out getting sunflower seeds and corn to fill their bellies. The difference from last year was startling. The beginning started with a heat wave, everything dry and drooping. Jimmy started with a bird feeder and water then. The birds and squirrels came to find the amazing food and water so needed.

The transformation thru the year to what I saw that day was striking. During that last year Jimmy had added to my Wildlife Garden to help the animals while inside the house he did things to help me through my treatment. As time went on he added two more bird feeders while trying to find foods to keep my body nourished and encourage eating. Then Jimmy added deer feeders to help them during the raging heat that killed all the forbs. Inside, Jimmy made sure I kept cool and entertained. Our AC went out, so he bought window units. He set up the TV with ways for me to watch movies.

As it moved into fall and winter Jimmy planted oats for the deer and bought me wigs to wear when I went in public and when I saw my grandkids. The view out my window had become a little peek into the wildlife world while inside feeling the warmth and love of Jimmy helping me through some of the toughest parts of my treatment.

As the new year approached I watched the rutting of the bucks and the beginning of the cycle of life to start again, for the fawns to be born the following spring. It was also the time of realization with my brain out of the fog. I could see the last of the year of treatments within sight. The joy that Jimmy and I could start talking and thinking and planning our future. To also see the cycle of our life would continue.

Then the wildflowers arrived with spring. The colors were abundant, and variety of flowers astounding. Jimmy added squirrel blocks and mowed the area to cut back the dead grass and give the forbs sunlight to grow. My body felt like the spring coming back to life. Jimmy bought me blouses to help me feel the recovery of my body back to normal. He was prepping the RV for our adventures we would start having again.

As I sat there looking out my window at the Wildlife Garden it was summer. It was the week that I would have my last infusion. This was the close of the year spent to conquer my breast cancer. The fawns were coming with their mothers. The tomato plants that I planted were growing fast and furiously. I was writing a book that I would never have thought was in my future. Jimmy and I were planning trips, talking about what we want to do the next year.

I saw the contrast from last year to the present in the Wildlife Garden, realizing the beauty of the growth and changes. Then I kept thinking about the contrast of our journey of going through all the phases of the roller coaster of killing cancer. It was always changing, never knowing exactly what would be around the next turn. Together we had handled everything as it changed. Together we kept strong and celebrated the progress along the way. I knew this week we would walk hand in hand out of the doctor's office to our car smiling. We would know that we had grown closer, enjoyed our time together this last year while completing the protocol of killing my breast cancer. It was amazing watching the Wildlife Garden grow and flourish while inside the same happened with us.

A year was a short time to make sure that Jimmy and I had a future. It had its times that were a bit trying and times when you couldn't help but laugh. Within everyone there is the ability to fight cancer especially with the encouragement of a partner, family and friends. It is something that is worth every minute and all your energy to battle.

Meeting with my oncologist, his favorite appointment of them all. He loved seeing me so animated. In fact, he said seeing his patients like this was his driving force. It may be our last appointment during treatment, yet not the end of the great relationship we had developed. We knew that my follow up appointments would be like visiting a friend. I could not thank him enough for being my oncologist and being straight with me on the climbing of each step of treatments.

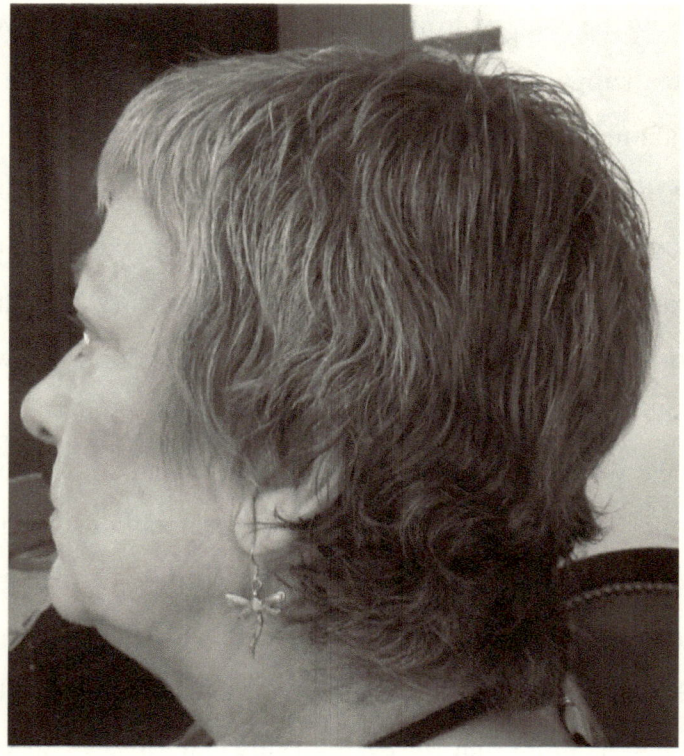

It had been Eight Months since my last chemotherapy, eight months of hair growth! I felt like I didn't look like a cancer patient anymore! WooHoo!

After the last infusion my plan included making an appointment with my hairdresser after the last infusion. I felt the time had come for me to get her help to make the changes for going forward to see myself in the mirror again and feel sexy.

Entering the infusion room for the last time is almost indescribable! I could not help but be excited! I know that is not a word that most people would use for walking into an infusion room, but it was for me. Knowing how quickly I would be crossing the finish line! Everyone was thrilled to be a part of the end. They too liked to see the patients with up-lifted spirits and share the feeling of accomplishment. Another wonderful addition, when my sister-in-law Jennifer and Megan our niece, stopped by on this final infusion. The hugs and congratulations were spectacular.

When we finished, Jimmy and I walked out with smiles and relief in our faces. All I wanted to do was get back to the ranch and spend the evening with Jimmy.

DONE!

All I kept thinking, the one word that covered that day. We had gone over the Speed Bump of Boob Cancer. The relief of having our world back seemed almost surrealistic. Jimmy and I had been through all the steps with goals at the end of each step. Knowing throughout this year that there is that final day at the end. We were there! We were DONE! We beat Boob Cancer! We did it together!

Jimmy had been my caregiver, friend, nurse, chef, protector, logistics manager and chauffeur. He had been very patient, kind, caring and loving during this whole process, more than anybody will ever know. With Jimmy by my side, the medical tools from my doctors and the knowledge that these were all I needed, I knew that Boob Cancer was doomed. I also had the love and support from all my family and friends. What more did I need? Just time to conquer!

It has been a journey that took us out of our norm. We had become so comfortable during this past fourteen months or so that it will be a change to get out of this recent feeling of norm. I had no doubt that it wouldn't take us long!

As I told my friends and family on social media I wanted to

thank everyone for their words of encouragement. The words had not been wasted. The breast cancer I had, (love saying "had") HER2-positive is so different and has made leaps and bounds in the medical field that I felt I had to share my story for others. Thanks to the family and friends that encouraged me to start writing this book after I finished chemotherapy. Now that I have finished the odyssey I will be able to finish the book. Unfortunately, there are no books on HER2-positive except text books. It has given me more of a reason to get it done quickly. I am writing the book to be the book I would have been very glad to have when I found out about my cancer. My hope is that it will give the reader a feeling of having a conversation with me about the whole experience.

I warned everyone on social media to get ready to see pictures of Jimmy and I getting back into adventures and events!

DONE! Not the end but the beginning!

Thoughts for You
Chapter 21

It has been eight months since the end of my chemotherapy treatments. My body has recovered in many ways, faster than I expected. In other ways I realize that it will be a year to get back to how I was before. Some of what Pollyanna Positive calls "future effects" are a bonus. The top of the effects to my future is that my legs have One-Tenth of the amount of hair than before! What a wonderful change! The effect of half as much hair in the crotch area is very apparent now. It seems that the hair growth under my left arm is half as much density as before. On the other hand, the hair growth under my right arm literally stops in a straight line halfway from before! If anybody had told me that there would be a straight cut-off line of my hair under my arm or anywhere, I would have thought, they were pulling my leg! The hair on my arms is the same thickness. Thank goodness my eyebrows came back, not as thick, they thinned after initially growing-in but some is better than none. Autumn has already found someone to do a henna fill of my eyebrows for me when I am ready. If the eyelashes had come back thicker that would have been great but they are the same as before. Oh well. The texture and look of my skin is much better. It had become thin, easily scratched, bleed, bruise, break out and chalky looking. Now it has returned to feel healthy and back to having color. The status of my fingernails is better. They seem to be growing out now though some seem to still be a little brittle. I have seen changes in my energy. The changes seem to be evident in three-week increments. Different chores I can do longer, and others are not stressful to do anymore. Occasionally I have a tired day for no reason. Jimmy always tells me not to fight it and rest. There is only one physical restriction, my right arm. I have trouble with some of the movement and especially stretching. It is the one the lymph node was taken from, which I have heard can be the reason. I know that with time and exercise it has and will continue to get better. The peripheral neuropathy is still present, but the numbness of my toes seems to be fifty percent less. The only physically visible leftover is the redness, warm and slight swelling of my boob from the radiation. Any thoughts of reconstruction surgery are not for now. I feel that in six months or more it will be enough time to consider what needs to be done, if anything, and my skin should be closer to normal. Remember there is not a specific time table.

As I mentioned in the beginning of the book, in situ is very important, stop it before it escapes. If every woman is responsible in getting mammograms the numbers of it being caught early would increase. It is something that every family should help their loved ones remember. I had not been responsible and then the death of my son Austin, I did not think of what I needed to do for myself. It added up to eight years of irresponsibility, that is such a Dangerously long time! I do not hesitate to remind women and ask them if they are up to date on their mammogram. So far, I have not offended anyone. If that happens, but they go get their mammogram, I am good with that.

When I learned that I had HER2-positive, I tried to find out anything and everything from anywhere or anyone. I talked with everyone I knew that had breast cancer. They all had the hormonal type. Research on the web was out of date on most of the websites. Knowing that I had to go through the treatments and had no clue what was going to happen was scary. If by writing this book, I hope I can help women who are faced with HER2-positive breast cancer and not feel so scary. It can help give the caregivers the vision needed to care for their loved ones.

The Window
Chapter 22

The positive attitude and determination are so important and is a must. They are part of seeing past the cancer. Seeing past the cancer for Jimmy and myself was "The Window." We both talked about what we would be able to do again and things that we wanted to do after we had conquered cancer. Imagine sitting at a window with images of your future. Our window kept changing as we progressed through the journey of Boob Cancer. Our favorite thing is to go camping in our RV to the Big Bend area. It has always been such a special place to get back to nature in the mountains. The magnificence of the energy that caused those beautiful mountains. The energy that has shaped them with the passage of time and weather. It is also very peaceful to be out away from the technology, the sounds of the busy world and all the distractions. To look up out there brings a sense of peace and awe with the beauty of the night sky filled with the brilliance of the stars and planets. The Rio Grande river adds the feeling of the flow of life that continues. I especially love it when it is monsoon season, which is during July through September in west Texas. The waterfalls created are extraordinary! For me it is the place I feel grounded.

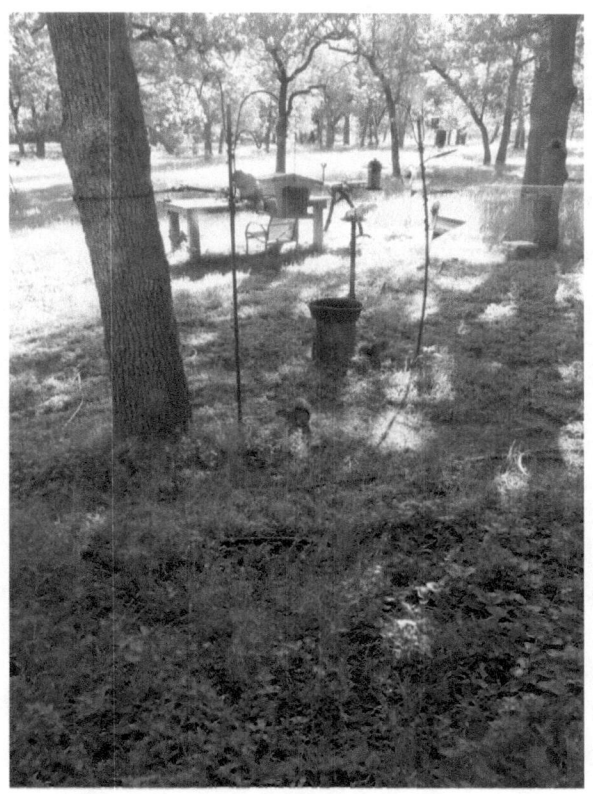

This is the inspirational view out my window.

The Window gave me a way to keep focused on the future. It is especially useful while handling the day-to-day trials, particularly during the chemotherapy. Take care, because all the steps can begin to consume your every thought every day. Jimmy always helped me to remember to see out the window at what our world would be after we conquered cancer. This journey wasn't one by choice, but one that we knew we could handle.

For all those patients with HER2-positive; my hope is that after reading this you will feel empowered with information to handle the treatments, confidence to know that each step is progress and assurance that you can conquer this cancer while having a positive attitude, determination and humor.

For all those caregivers; my hope is that after reading you will understand what your love one may experience. You need to help them keep the positive attitude to get thru all the steps. You need to help them keep track of all their appointments and get them there. You need to keep all the receipts, instructions, bills and payments. You also need to just love them.

For those who are medical staff; my hope is that you now have a peek into what the patient and caregivers are going through when you see them. Remember that they have worked hard when you meet them or since the last time you saw them. No matter your job, in whatever step they are in, it is but a part of the whole process they are experiencing. Many of the medical staff I met during my process of all the steps never knew what else the patients experienced. I hope that I have given you some knowledge to understand your patient a little bit better.

www.ingramcontent.com/pod-product-compliance
Lightning Source LLC
Chambersburg PA
CBHW020243290526
45784CB00003B/1085